Other works by Christine Holubec-Jackson:

7 Jars of Hot Pickled Peppers: A Roller Coaster Ride to Acceptance
ISBN: 978-1-7753999-1-9

The Adventures of Glia Girl: When Stroke Strikes
ISBN: 978-17753999-3-3

The Adventures of Glia Girl: Ouch!
ISBN: 978-1-7753999-5-7

I AM ALIVE

My Journey To, Through, and Beyond Strokes and Brain Surgery!

CHRISTINE HOLUBEC-JACKSON

I AM ALIVE

This book is a memoir. Although some events have been compressed the author has done her best to accurately reflect her memories and experiences over time. Efforts have been made to ensure any information offered is accurate and correct. The author accepts no liability for error and takes no responsibility for loss or damage because of a person doing something in response to information provided in this book. This book does not provide legal or lifestyle change advice, and the reader should always seek professional advice from a healthcare professional or personal therapist prior to making any personal changes.

Published by Christine Holubec-Jackson, Edmonton, Canada

Copyright: 1206091

ISBN:
    Paperback   978-1-775-3999-8-8
        ebook   978-1-775-3999-9-5

Publication assistance by

PAGEMASTER
PUBLISHING
PageMaster.ca

Dedication

Contents

*"What a precious privilege it is to be alive. To breathe,
to think, to enjoy, to love." Marcus Aurelius*

I

Introduction:

Phone calls with loved ones, caring, compassionate texts and messages, help from an aide to straighten my blankets. So much kindness. Everyone's love and care envelopes and protects me, like a warm, soft cloak wrapped around my shoulders, keeping out the worst of the raging winter blizzard. It's woven with love, strength, prayers, and positive energy. With my cloak of care firmly in place I can heal. I can move forward, do what I need to do and be who I need to be.

People are so kind in their words, so generous in their support and actions. It surrounds me and reaches down to touch my soul. There is no choice. With so much love I can't help but improve and get better. I must try my hardest, give it my all. One step at a time, to get stronger and gain back my independence just so I have an opportunity to give back to all these amazing people; to have a chance to pay it forward to anyone who needs a smile, a helping hand, a prayer, or a candle lit.

That's my choice, but it's really not a choice. It's like a healthy baby, thriving, loved, and well cared for; cherished. They don't make a choice when they start to sit up, roll over, crawl, walk. It's just the way it is. The natural succession of growing and learning. Some take to it faster than others, but they are milestones achieved by most.

That's me; it's just the way it is. Soon I'll be sitting, then standing, then walking again with my cloak of love and support helping me every step of the way. My success belongs to all who have helped to weave the fabric. I know I am not alone. I am forever grateful. I want to succeed so I can be in a place where I have the honour of being a thread in someone else's cloak.

"Inhale, exhale, it is well, it is well. All of this is
part of the story you will tell." Anonymous

PROLOGUE:

It's been four years, 1 month and 25 days since I first found out I had bleeding in my brain. Four years, 1 month and 25 days and here I am again. Sitting in the hospital with a doctor telling me my brain is bleeding. Maybe I should have expected it. They hadn't been able to repair it the first two times around.

The first time, four years and change ago, my brain started bleeding from an abnormality called a cavernous malformation. There were several of these little malformations, described as blackberries in the pons area of my brain stem. They were being fed by veins and may have been there my entire life. Why one of them decided to start bleeding, causing me to have a stroke, we'll never know. That's just life.

The pons area of the brain stem is in a tricky location. It is referred to as the superhighway of the brain as all the information needed for thinking and for sustaining life goes through it. Four years ago, the area was inoperable. But luck was on my side, and it stopped bleeding on its own. Lucky that I was still alive, not so lucky that it left me with some permanent disabilities. But, luckily again, most were manageable.

I could think, I could talk, and, with lots of hard work, I could walk. I had incredible support from a program called S-ESD, Stroke, Early Supported Discharge. I had a whole team of stroke specialized therapists come to my home, almost every day for five weeks, providing me with much needed rehabilitation to support me in my recovery. I had so much help and most important, I was alive! Yes, very lucky.

The event was life altering for me. So much so, I wrote a book about my experience. The subtitle was "A Roller Coaster Ride to Acceptance". How naive I was back then. I recently reread my book. The entire book was redolent of my desire to return to work. By the end of the book, I was still only in the early acceptance phase of my journey. I was learning but I hadn't fully come to terms with what it meant to be a stroke survivor and live with a brain injury. I thought I'd be returning to my old life, my old self, maybe even my promotion at work. Was work really such a prized part of my life?

At that time, it was. I had had a few career changes and this last job, well, it was the one! I loved it. I worked in metallurgy, testing steel. Mostly I did ultrasonic testing on steel grinding rods, used for crushing raw material in mining, but I could do all the different analyses, using the mass spectrometer, microhardness of spring steel, determining the yield and rupture point of rebar. I worked hard and it paid off.

The same day I found out my brain was bleeding, the exact same day, I was offered a promotion at work. If that's not irony, I don't know what is. There was a lesson to be learned for sure. Maybe life isn't all about work and perceived success; work is not our identity. The stroke sure pushed my life in a different direction, but I believe it was the path I was supposed to follow. And follow it I did, trying to make the best out of that unimaginable situation.

Work and family were the two most important parts of my life. My husband, Ken, and I had a solid marriage built on trust, respect, love, and compassion. We had three beautiful children together. At the time of my stroke, our eldest daughter, Kaylyn, was living up north and working in her chosen career, environmental education, and conservation.

Our son, Kevin, had two degrees under his belt, music and education. He was embarking on two new adventures. One was to get his master's degree in music and the other was to marry the love of his life, Alix. She had the same two degrees as Kevin and was fully supportive of Kevin's desire to further his education and passion for music. They were planning to move to Vancouver over the summer, where he would be attending university, in the fall.

Our youngest, our baby Emily, was finishing her last year of high school. She had applied to university and would be attending in the fall. Who knew what life adventures she would be embarking upon? My family, my children were paramount in my life. I love them beyond compare. I also tried to balance life as a mother with full-time employment.

Life has a way of presenting us with situations that push us in a new direction. Sometimes the signs of life are gentle and nudging. Other times they are a BRIDGE OUT AHEAD leaving you no choice but to change course. The stroke washed out the bridge on the highway of my life. I was on a new path.

The events that led me to becoming employed at a steel mill were somewhere in between nudging and Bridge Out, edging closer to the washed-out bridge. I was all in, a "lifer" in my previous career. Events that are too outrageous to even imagine altered my life trajectory. I won't go into too many details, but it involved trying to handle the aftermath of a workplace murder. I was in a senior management position and a lot of the responsibility came to me.

I was managing a program for people with complex disabilities. One such client had very complex challenges, none of them his own fault. He was born into a life and family that could not support him and was maybe even complicit in his challenges. We had had a prior incident that was foreshadowing to the murder that had me sitting in a hospital room, with two RCMP officers and this client, awaiting his transfer to a secure facility that could manage his behaviours.

The young man was no longer in our care when the murder occurred, but we had provided the most care for him historically. The police came to our organization for answers for how this could happen. I was involved in police interviews. Reports I had written were entered into evidence. A few co-workers were also called in for questioning. I tried to be there for them. The person murdered was a relative of one of my leadership team. It was inconceivable that I attended the funeral of the person who was murdered by another person I had spent eight years trying to support. Truth is so much stranger than fiction.

Once the dust had settled, I had nothing left. I was empty. I resigned, taking a leap of faith, not knowing what was next but knowing I could not continue where I was. Help came to me in the form of a job at the steel mill. I barely knew what I was applying for, nor what the job would entail. Luckily, they were as desperate for employees as I was for a new career and thus started a new chapter.

I had a background in chemistry but otherwise I was as green as they come. I used to love the show, "Grizzly Adams". The old trapper always called Grizzly Adams a "green horn" referring to how ill-equipped Adams was to live in the wilderness. Adams did pretty good and so did I in the steel mill. I had found my niche.

As I got to know the job and the steel mill better, I was able to move into a position that no longer required twelve-hour shift work. I never got used to night shifts. I had asked one seasoned employee if night shifts still bothered him. He looked me straight in the eye and said after 32 years he still hated them!

There were opportunities available and soon I became the workplace First Aid Instructor, on top of my regular job. I had taught First Aid in my previous workplace and had been an instructor for over twenty years. Teaching at the steel mill was so interesting. Being a high hazard industry, along with twelve-hour shift work for many, brought a real feeling of camaraderie. I had fun teaching every course and many employees discovered their latent acting talent when we did simulated scenarios.

Another opportunity I had was to be part of a focus group to encourage more women into non-traditional roles. We met several times and partnered with a group that provided apprenticeships to women in trades. Once, I volunteered at the Edmonton Women's Show. It was so much fun talking to different women about working in a steel mill, although many of their husbands seemed more interested.

I embraced my desire to expand people's thoughts towards career choices. My son Kevin's fiancée, Alix, was working as a kindergarten teacher, having just graduated from university, a temporary position before their move to Vancouver. She graciously let me come in and talk to the kiddies about what I did. My company supported this opportunity, arming me with pens, stickers and note pads to give out. I brought my hard hat and some steel samples. It was a great time and maybe one of them will grow up to consider metallurgy as a career.

One of my biggest opportunities came in the form of covering for a paternity leave in a supervisory position in shipping.

The steel mill shipped out many, many tons of steel every day. It travelled by truck or railcar. There was a crew of about nineteen people who worked 24/7, stacking bundles of steel, checking loads and filling orders, using two overhead magnetic gantry cranes. I thrived in this job and the crew were very helpful. They were the experts, and I was excited to learn from them. One veteran employee, nicknamed Raspy, knew shipping better than anyone and was pleased to have someone listen to his commonsense approach for loading the steel and filling orders.

Once the paternity leave ended, I returned to my regular position but still covered when needed. I found the job challenging and fulfilling. It was the right time in my life to take on such a role as well. There were rumours that the regular supervisor was trying for another position. I was hopeful, not only would I be the one of the few female supervisors in operations, but it would also include a good pay raise. This was the promotion I was offered the day I found out my brain was bleeding for the first time. Thus started my detour in the rollercoaster ride of surviving a stroke.

"Life is a journey, not a destination. The memories we gather along the way are the treasures of our travels." CHJ

CHAPTER 1

THE NEW JOURNEY:

It's funny. When you look back the timeline of events is laid out in such an even, chronological order. This event led to another and so on. It seems like a straight line from cause to affect. In reality, the way is filled with twists and turns, just like the proverbial roller coaster. When we're in the thick of it, living it, it is difficult to see tomorrow's effects from today's actions.

Since my first stroke, life has been topsy turvy. Not only for me but for my entire family. Here is an observation of what I wish we could have done from reflecting on the past: we should have all gone for family counselling. This is one regret I will carry forever as my stroke affected my entire family. My husband was there for me, so supportive but each of my children was affected differently. One more instance of the line being straight when we look back but too convoluted to see what's next when we look towards the future.

A dear friend of mine and I had recently reconnected after a number of years. She and her husband had moved away. Far away, right across the country. When we first moved to Wetaskiwin, we started a running club together. We called ourselves "The Wetaskiwin Road Runners". It was so much fun, and our highlight was organizing a yearly relay marathon from another small city to ours. The grand prize for the event was a free team entry for the Canadian Death Race. A crazy race, covering 125 kilometers through the mountains. I ran twice in the Death Race, as part of a team. We also taught running boot camps and had fun hosting the annual Red Dress Run and Turkey Trot.

After my friend and her husband moved, she started her own wellness and personal coaching business. We reconnected three years after my first stroke. After our visit she wanted to do an article on her website about my personal journey. I was honoured that she considered my story worth sharing. In preparation she sent me a few questions to answer. One of my answers included my remorse over not having sought out family counselling.

My family paid the price for this omission. I had always thought we were strong, grounded, and would always be there for each other. Any life-altering event affects more than just the person who experienced it. I often say that it is easier to bear hardship yourself than watch someone you love go through it. I was so headstrong in my own recovery and still good friends with denial. I forgot about my family.

PODCASTS

I was searching so hard for my new identity without my career. My husband was always there for me, always trying to help. Initially, Ken organized for me to be a guest on some radio shows, talking about my experience and trying to spread information about stroke. These seemed positive and despite how nervous I was I found it fulfilling.

Then Ken suggested he and I start a podcast. I barely knew what podcasts were, let alone conduct one myself. The idea was ignited by one of Kevin's friends who had visited over Christmas after my first stroke. I was still searching for my identity, looking for something to fill the hole by my loss of career. I was also trying to make the most out of my time. I was getting used to living with the malformation in my brain stem, but it was kind of like living with a sword over my head.

This young man did a weekly podcast himself. I was learning Twitter, trying to post something stroke related daily, but I wanted to do more, I just didn't know what. I had been considering starting a blog. Suddenly a podcast seemed like a great way to reach people. It had the added benefit that it was something Ken and I could do together. My goal was to help others: I wanted other survivors to know they weren't alone.[1]

Ken and I really didn't know what we were doing but we learned together. We were still trying to muddle through managing my life altering stroke. One of the ways we knew how was by creating and building endeavours to work on together. Ken took care of all the recording, sound and editing. Thank goodness. He was excited to learn more about recording and sound files. Ken always had a gift for the technical side of sound, doing all the sound setup for our band.

Have I mentioned Ken and I are in a band together? I play bass and he plays the drums. Ken is the band manager, and we have three other members who have become like family. I started learning bass about ten years ago, on Ken's suggestion, so we could spend more time together. He's been a drummer practically all his life. Thus started our band. I loved it and was able to return to it after my stroke. It was different just like everything else in my life but at least I could still play well enough to be a part of it.

For the podcasts, I wrote the monologue and interview questions. It was all about stroke or surviving any life altering event. We were trying to spread information and inspiration. We were so blessed with every guest who agreed to be interviewed, sharing their experiences, expertise, insights, and inspiration. My goal aligned with all our guests, to help others and let other survivors of stroke or any life altering event know they weren't alone.

My first experience of realizing I wasn't alone had come from the most surprising place. Our niece, Ken's brother's daughter, was participating in a rehabilitation program in Edmonton. Ken's brother lived in Saskatchewan, and she had no one else nearby. We offered to drive up for a visit, let her know some family was not too far away.

---

1   The name of our podcast series is: 7 Jars of Hot Pickled Peppers. You can find it through our website or on Podbean, iTunes and on YouTube.)

Several years back Ken's niece suffered a tragic accident that caused a traumatic brain injury. We had given what support we could at the time, distance limiting our involvement. Meeting her again now, after my own brain injury was a breakthrough moment for me. Despite the vastly different mechanisms for the bleeding in our brains, we shared a number of similar effects. It was so comforting to talk to someone who got it, who could understand my symptoms completely with minimal explanation. We bonded over our shared challenges and developed a kinship that will last forever. It really helped me along my road to acceptance back then.

One of our initial podcasts was with Ken's niece. She was able to share her story and we were able to promote the fact that a stroke is a brain injury. This was something I never considered before. Equating stroke with brain injury really helped me to find more compassion for myself. The first few podcasts were flavoured with my desire to understand my own journey and accept my new normal.

Ken took care of all the technical parts of the podcasts while I wrote the outline. Ken also took care of organizing interviews with various guests. Another of our inaugural podcasts featured my sister, Cami. Cami had been instrumental during my stroke as she was a nurse practitioner whose celebrated career included working with neurology and stroke.

With her we did an interview where she defined the different types of strokes. When I first had mine, I was in disbelief that I had even had a stroke. Just admitting to being a stroke survivor was difficult. She helped me to come to terms with stroke and educated all of us about stroke in general as well as specifics to mine. There was no one better suited to help our potential listeners understand the multiple layers entrenched within that one, encompassing word – STROKE!

Cami lived in Niagara Falls. It added another layer of technical challenge for Ken to figure out in recording our interview. He had the hard work; Cami and I had a lot of laughs trying to figure out how to do the interview successfully over the phone, as well as trying to control our nervousness. Ken still says that interview had the most editing of any of them. She completed another one with us, where she described the different types of vertigo. Again, this was something that explained one of my own challenges, my ongoing dizziness.

Creating and producing our podcasts was the pinnacle to my recovery and really helped me come to terms with my new normal. We were trying to spread information and inspiration. Along with Cami and Ken's niece, we had three different neurologists, stroke therapists, stroke and traumatic brain injury survivors, a quilting expert, even a rock star. Every time someone agreed to do a podcast with us, I was so humbled by their generous gift of time. Their generosity helped me immensely in my mission to give back while discovering my new normal.

Ken and I were so busy with completing podcasts. I was still trying to recover from my stroke. When I listen to those podcasts, I hear my voice and the struggles I sometimes had with my speech. My time was limited by my energy level. As much as I was busy, I also needed lots of time for rest. Fatigue after any brain injury can be substantial. It seemed as if I was on the go all the time but really, I only spent a few hours a week on the podcasts.

When I go back and listen to our first podcasts, I laugh. We were so green and new to it. After our first season I was doing much better. Kevin was instrumental in helping us, creating accompanying YouTube videos for the recordings. He did a fantastic job and all while completing his Masters' degree.

MEMOIR

Another project that occupied my time was writing, self-publishing and then promoting my first memoir. "7 Jars of Hot Pickled Peppers; A Roller Coaster Ride to Acceptance." It's quite a title and so named due to my love of hot pickled peppers. It is one of the few foods I can taste since stroke took most of my sense of taste. The memoir started out as a journal of my recovery. Ken brought me a beautiful journal while I was still in the hospital and encouraged me to write down my progress.

My journal became my memoir. As I was writing the bulk of it, I realized I had eaten seven big jars of hot pickled peppers. Hence the name. Again, it seemed as if we were very busy, but it was such a different type of busy and the days are long when you are recovering from a life-altering event.

When I look back at it, I see the raw and honest account of my journey as a young stroke survivor. An interesting fact: if you have a stroke before age sixty-five, you are considered young. As I mentioned earlier, it really focused on my loss of career and my hope of returning to work. The end of the book is a true testament to my lack of understanding of the life altering effects of stroke. It clearly showcased my desire, my expectation, to return to my old life.

I still thought, somehow, someway, I would return to it. There is no old life. There is just my life, here and now. I was learning more each day and the excitement of promoting my book helped with accepting the changes stroke wrought, the acceptance that was missing when I penned my journey. It was and still is a fair representation of the initial phase of my journey towards true acquiescence. We all have the responsibility of creating a loop between who we were to who we are. It's a lifelong journey and every change challenges us to join who we were to who we are.

Ken, my biggest supporter and promoter, organized several book signings at "Chapters/Indigo" bookstores. It was usually pretty quiet, and we discovered that my book title was misleading. Many people thought it was a cookbook. To help with the misconception, Ken developed a bookmark with the stroke acronym FAST on the back. FAST represents the best way to recognize and manage a suspected stroke. It also highlights the importance of quick treatment; Time is Brain! Perhaps I should have changed the name to be more accurate about my stroke journey, but I've stuck to my guns and it's even my Twitter handle, @7jars.

The book signings were usually quiet with only mild interest. That was until one day my friend, Joan, took me. She has missed her calling as a salesperson or maybe a preacher. Joan could sell the proverbial ice cubes to a penguin. We talked to so many people and sold lots of books. It was a thrilling day. Not only my good friend but also my advocate and biggest promoter. It seemed when Joan was with me, I sold lots of books and was able to spread my message. We didn't make any money, but the sales went a long way towards helping us to cover our costs.

Joan and I had been friends for a long time. Before my stroke we had some great adventures. In the winter we would often go cross-country skiing. Usually, cross country skiers follow a nicely laid track along beautiful snowy trails. Not us. We broke our own trail along the ravine behind her acreage. It followed a creek, thankfully frozen over during the winter.

One time we went on a clear, full moon night. It was beautiful, and a little eerie, especially when a large owl flew by. Another time, my son, Kevin, came with us. Always the dare devil, he skied or climbed up the sides of the ravine to jump into huge snow drifts. That's why when we skied on a warm day at the end of winter, we made Kevin ski across the creek first. We were sure the ice would hold him...

I thought of Joan first when I was invited to speak at a local library in a nearby community. Ken was busy so I asked Joan if she could take me. I had gotten my driver's license back since my first stroke, but I really only drove in town and never at night. The library talk was in the evening and out of town. Joan not only drove me, but she also brought another one of our friends along.

It was a great time. I had changed my delivery, trying to get my message out and included reading a small passage from my book. There was an added benefit to this talk. It was a small group from a small community, and we were able to have some open discussion after. It was very meaningful to me. I am always so humbled that anyone would want to read my words or listen to me speak, let alone find them helpful within their own lives. I was and am so grateful anytime sharing my experiences can aid someone else.

With Joan there that night, we celebrated selling the rest of the books I had. I was so excited. We had covered most of the costs of self-publishing and had a little extra to get some more books printed. My goal was never to make money, both Ken and I were realistic about that. Maybe it's all those years I spent working for Not-for-Profit agencies. The book, the podcasts, all were done with the intent to help others and give back.

In the midst of podcasts and promoting my book, Kevin and his love, Alix were married. It was a beautiful wedding. A time of family, friends, and a celebration of their love. I was so happy for them. I was so grateful that despite all the life changes imparted from stroke, I was still alive and able to be there with them and for them.

I was finding my new purpose in life and perhaps even some calm within the maelstrom of stroke survival. Along with our podcasts I was writing a newsletter that I shared virtually. Again, I mostly focused on stroke recovery. I was very headstrong. I really feel it got me through the tough times, kept me going and pushed me to do what I could within my new limits. As much as I tried to help others, I didn't pay enough attention to my own family and their feelings.

FAMILY and ANOTHER BLEED

Never again will I take any relationship for granted as I watched my family go through some very difficult times, including mental health concerns and creating distance, needing space. I know we cannot live in the past; we need to live for today, plan for tomorrow, but I would endure many more strokes to be able to go back in time and do things differently. Everything happens for a reason although I haven't figured this one out yet.

Our eldest daughter, Kaylyn, told us she needed a break from the family, and it continues, even as I write this. This happened after she eloped with her girlfriend. On Christmas Eve, about a year and a half after my stroke, she told us she and her girlfriend were married already; six months prior. They had secretly married three days before Kevin and Alix's wedding. We were so confused. They had a wedding planned, a date one year in the future, they had even asked for my help with different parts of the wedding and the whole time they were already married. I was devastated.

We were trying to repair ourselves from this announcement when our youngest daughter, Emily, opened up to us about her own struggles with mental health. We tried our best to support her and find her the help she needed. Shortly thereafter, the distance our Kaylyn felt she needed increased. I'll never fully understand but I hold onto the hope that she has done what she feels is best for her and is living her best life. It is this thought that keeps me from completely succumbing to my broken heart.

The true definition of family exceeds just blood relations. It's the time, love, support, sharing and caring that count, that's what makes family. I am very blessed to have many people I call family. But I was desperate for my own little circle of my husband and our children to be together, to be a healthy unit. It was in earnest that the most important advice I could offer about my journey when my friend wrote her blog was to remember your whole family is affected when you go through a life altering event. I tried hard to keep these devastating emotions locked up and appreciate the people in my life who love me, brain injury and all.

When things first started falling apart with my family, I was so desperate to find some kind of balm for this wound that I worked myself up into a tizzy, causing another, small bleed. It was still in that inoperable location but luckily minor enough not to need treatment. It was significant enough to cause me a few more challenges, including my speech, my walking, and my driving. Worst, it dashed away any hope of returning to work. I cringed when my doctor wrote "permanently disabled" on my medical report.

As much as I was expecting it, the diagnosis still carried a shock. The risk I carried was predominant in our lives and why would I do anything to aggravate it? My old friend Denial and I still had a strong relationship. Work is inherent to stress; it is not all bad but it "comes with the job!" I couldn't manage the drive just to get to work, let alone the pressures of timelines, multiple meetings, computer work, problem solving, the list goes on. All the things that fed and excited me about work now were my nemesis towards causing that little malformation in my head to wreak havoc to my life, perhaps even take my life.

There is a bright side to this tale. The latest brain bleed introduced me to my neurosurgeon who would become an extremely important part of my life two years in the future. He took over my care from my neurologist. At that time, monitoring the malformation was the best treatment option, with regular MRI's. Surgery was just too risky. We were slowly learning to live with a sword over our head, never knowing when it might drop.

MENTAL HEALTH

Once I had recuperated enough and knowing we needed help recovering from all the mayhem, Ken sought out a psychologist for us to see, together. We had faced my stroke and two of our children's mental health challenges together. We would heal together as well.

There is some stigma surrounding reaching out for mental health help. I grew up in a family where we took care of our problems privately. We were very practical; we took things in stride and handled it. I was embarrassed to share some of our difficulties but pleasantly surprised at the understanding and helping hands from my parents and sisters once I was brave enough to reveal the mental health challenges with ourselves and our daughters. They only offered support and love. We got the same response from the friends we shared with.

It was and is an essential lesson for all of us. Mental health concerns should be treated with as much conviction and support as any physical ailment. Many years ago, when I had just started working at the steel mill, my older cousin committed suicide. We weren't super close, as she lived in Toronto, but we did keep in touch, sending regular letters. I had just sent one for her fiftieth birthday and had received a very nice response. I thought she was okay. The family knew she had some challenges, but no one recognized the depth of her need. It was heartbreaking. Now I was learning the lesson anew.

Not only was I discovering the importance of asking for help with my physical recovery from stroke, but I was also learning that it is okay to need help with the emotional, psychological side of life altering events. We all need to be kind and understanding, especially to ourselves. I wish I had more insight all those years ago. Both for my cousin and my own plight when dealing with the workplace murder. Life and learning just takes time. I was nervous but looking forward to meeting with the psychologist.

If this was a Hallmark movie, we would have all made-up and been a perfect family unit again, ready to face the challenges of life and stroke. We were so wrong. Our life was about to hit the "mindbender" of roller coaster rides, the name of the iconic roller coaster in West Edmonton Mall, at that time, the world's largest indoor triple loop roller coaster.

We met with our psychologist, the first time I had ever done anything like this, for me. She was kind, compassionate and very knowledgeable. She helped us to realize how much we had been through; we were still going through. The two hours flew by. We shared our challenges, some tears and left with a book to read and a feeling of hope that as bad as things were, they were going to get better. We went to bed feeling lighter, our problems weighing a little less on our hearts.

Then it all crashed in!!!

"You, me, or nobody is gonna hit as hard as life. But it ain't how hard you hit; it's about how hard you can get hit and keep moving forward. How much you can take and keep moving forward." Rocky Balboa

CHAPTER 2

THE INCIDENT

Buzz, buzz, buzz. I dizzily turned over in bed. Turning in bed is challenging as I still slept on an incline. Sleeping flat on my back exacerbated my vertigo too much. What was that noise? I managed to turn towards my nightstand. My phone vibrated on my night table, having set it on silent for the night. I grabbed it, hearing Ken starting to stir beside me. Squinting from the bright screen I tried to focus my eyes. They still didn't work quite right since my first stroke. Our RING doorbell was telling me there was someone at the door. What? It was the middle of the night. I opened the app and saw an RCMP officer at our door, at 3:30 in the morning!

I sat up in bed and loudly told Ken, "There's a police officer at our door!" Ken sat straight up. He quickly got dressed. I pulled on a housecoat. By the time we got to the door, the RCMP officer had left. We looked out, wondering what was going on. I immediately thought of our children; were they all okay? Holding onto the railing for balance and support, I went downstairs and onto our driveway. Ken was looking across the street. Our neighbour was standing in his driveway. He was pointing behind us, at our garage door.

It was surreal, things like this only happen in movies, horror movies. We turned around and gasped. Our driveway, our garage door, and Ken's work vehicle were covered in graphic, hateful graffiti. I stood, dumbfounded. Ken was in shock and looked back to our neighbour, now coming over. Just as our neighbour started to explain what was going on, the police came back.

We listened in disbelief as the events of the last hour unfolded. Our neighbours' wife woke up to tend to their young daughter. She glanced outside and noticed two young men in hoodies committing the atrocious acts on our property. She woke up her husband and then tried to take a photo of the crime. I'll never forget when she described how the young men noticed her in the window, looked up, smiled, and just slowly started walking away. It just sends shivers throughout my body.

Her husband, in an act of protective bravery, dashed out of their house, baseball bat in hand while she called 911 for the police. I feel sick when I think about what could have happened and am so grateful that the perpetrators fled as our neighbour chased them. He returned, unscathed, and the police continued the chase. The criminals were nowhere to be found.

Ken and I didn't know what to say. On closer inspection of the horrible, spraypainted scrawls, it seemed a death threat was implied between the gang signs and vulgar icons. As we looked around, we discovered that the graffiti continued into our backyard, covering the side of our house. How had we not heard anything?

They were in our backyard! We felt violated. It seemed the event was a targeted attack against Ken. He was a Federal Parole Officer and worked for Canada Services Corrections. His job entailed regular meetings with offenders that had served federal prison time once they were released. Ken ran a satellite office, right in our home. He never met offenders at our house, always meeting them at their work or their home, sometimes the coffee shop. Ken always told our friends, "If you see me at Tim Horton's with someone you don't know, walk away." We lived in a small city, around 14,000 people. We couldn't help but occasionally run into his clients.

Usually, that didn't matter. These were people who had served their time and were trying to make the best of a new life. Lately though, things had changed and several of Ken's clients were gang members. I don't know too much about gangs but there seemed to be a different level of violence and a loyalty to the gang that surpassed any common sense or reasoning. We were witnessing it firsthand. Ours was the only house defiled in the neighbourhood. Ken's work vehicle, the one he used for all his meetings with offenders, was grossly coated; no other vehicle was touched.

In speaking with the police officers, they felt it was an attack, whether against Ken personally or against Corrections Canada, who knew? They recognized the threat. One officer candidly told us to keep a baseball bat handy and be ready to protect ourselves. He went on to say not to use guns, as we could be charged if we shot someone but with a bat it would be seen as self-defense. The officer also included that it was better to kill any perpetrator, again, as long as it was in self-defense.

I was in disbelief. Never, in my wildest imagination (and I have an extremely vivid imagination) did I ever consider that we could have this type of conversation, on our driveway at 4:00 in the morning; talking about inflicting injury onto someone else because that person wanted to hurt us. Suddenly understanding stroke and brain injury seemed a whole lot easier than trying to comprehend the senseless madness these thugs imparted. The officers both believed the two perpetrators were low level gang members trying to build some "cred" (credibility) within the gang.

The police also believed that there was little hope of ever apprehending them. Their own resources were stretched thin with more need than capacity. Ken had mentioned maybe they could get fingerprints from the spray cans that they left lying around. Their crime lab was also lacking in resources and even if they did find usable fingerprints, they probably wouldn't stand up in court anyway. Sometimes I think our system protects the criminal more than the victim. It sure wasn't anything like those crime shows on TV.

The police left saying they would be in touch. Ken, in his role, was a Peace Officer and he often worked collaboratively with the RCMP. This was an affront to one of their own. They felt outraged by the attack as well. They would be keeping an extra watchful eye on us and our neighbourhood. Ken was on the phone with the on-call center of the head office in

Ottawa, but by now it was only 5:00 AM and a Saturday morning. Then we discovered something even worse.

We went into the garage, getting supplies to clean off Ken's work vehicle. There had been heavy dew that night and we thought we could scrub and wash most of the spray paint off the car. We had taken multiple photos, as had the police, and we wanted to erase the awful graphics as soon as possible.

That's when we saw it. The gang members had been in our attached garage. They had sat in our vehicles parked inside. They had gone through our glove boxes, taken out our registration and insurance. They had been looking for whose house it was. There was no doubt now that this was targeted, whether against Ken or Federal Corrections, we'll never know. They had been one door away from being inside our house. Ken and I looked at each other, horror in our eyes. There were no words to express the unfathomable fear of what could have happened. We contacted the police again. They came, wrote another statement, and took even more photos.

Our home, our refuge from the world, was no longer safe. My brain injured mind was having troubles taking it all in. So, I resorted to what I did best, I focused on one thing and one thing only. My recovery had taught me this. We even did a podcast episode about it. Sometimes you need to focus on one tree, not the whole forest.

The car was our first tree to focus on. We were able to wash most of the spray paint off, erasing the ugliness. If only we could erase the vicious malice the graffiti represented from our hearts as quickly as we had from the car. I helped more than I should have, knowing I would pay for it later, but I felt I had no other choice. We had to get rid of the physical signs as soon as possible.

Removing the defacements from our house, garage door and driveway presented more of a challenge. The sun was up, and it was going to be a beautiful, sunny, and warm summer day. This seemed so incongruous with how we were feeling. By this time, Ken had spoken to the on-call headquarters in Ottawa and then the District Director. There was a general reaction of shock. Not once had this ever happened to another Parole Officer, in all of Canada.

THE AFTERMATH

There had been untoward comments to Parole Officers, even delving into threats, but these officers worked in office buildings, had their meetings there, and returned to their anonymous homes after work. They didn't have a work vehicle parked in front of their house. This knowledge brought us no comfort, instead elevated our unease. Ken's employers were trying to be as supportive as possible, but this was unchartered territory, for everyone. We were offered multiple times the chance to stay in a hotel, Ken's work covering the expenses.

We seriously considered it. But this was our home. We were not going to be scared off or bullied to leave. We were going to stay, we were going to clean up the desecration, we were going to fight for what was right. This was our home, our life. Ken told his employer we were staying. Little did we realize how difficult the coming days and months were going to be.

By mid-morning some neighbours had come over to help clean, one bringing us donuts and drinks. Our youngest daughter, Emily, also came and lent her elbow grease. She was currently living in a basement suite, close to where she was going to university. Soon we noticed a string of vehicles slowly driving down our little side street. Ours was a quiet neighbourhood with limited traffic. Word travelled fast and people wanted to come see first-hand the vandalism that rocked our peaceful part of town.

The cleaning was challenging, with the paint stubbornly clinging to the sides of our house and garage. The sun had baked it on. There was no way to clean the paint off the driveway, so Ken found some old grey paint and covered it up. It would take several more coats, more paint than we had. There continued to be a faint outline of a caricatured male body part spewing all over the driveway, until we could purchase more paint.

Some more of our dear friends came by later and with them brought a miracle cleaner. He worked for the school district and regularly they had to clean off graffiti from their buildings. He brought their cleaner and it worked incredibly well. We all wore rubber gloves and had a pile of rags. I couldn't keep up with the work, stroke preventing me from helping as much as I would have liked. Our friends knew my limits and cheerfully carried on cleaning while encouraging me to rest.

We ordered pizza for supper, even having some laughs while we worked together. Underlying the camaraderie inspired by the shared work was the feeling of dread and concern for our safety. Our friends left, most of the mess was purged from the outside of our house. A quiet stillness descended on our house. It should have been peaceful, but it was anything but. Without the busyness of work and other people our fear and anxiety climbed to new heights.

That night was the worst. Neither Ken nor I slept. We were scared, overwhelmed, over-tired, in shock. The gravity of the situation was still sinking in. The saying goes that God won't give you more than you can handle but our limits were surely being tested. Ken turned very intense, trying to clean up the rest of the mess, and keep us as safe as possible. Unreasonably, he felt it was his fault. Regrettably, situations like these don't contain a lot of common sense. It mirrored my own feelings that somehow my stroke was my fault. Both of our thoughts of blame were absurd. His work tried to support him, us, in this abhorrent act and offered to have an alarm system installed for our house.

FULL UP

It wasn't enough. After the alarm system was installed and all traces of the graffiti erased, the wounds of the event weren't healing. Ken was doubting his work decisions and every time we saw someone in a hoodie or gang tags in town, it would trigger the event all over again. Ken didn't want to leave me in the house alone at all and would call often, checking up on me and ensuring I had everything locked up tight when he had to leave for work meetings. Ken ensured our house was super safe and we were ready to protect ourselves. There were baseball bats in every corner and pepper spray tucked in nooks. He ordered hunting knives that he hid in various places. We took a trip to a sporting goods store that specialized in batons fashioned with tasers on one end. Ken bought two. Every night he triple-checked all the doors and alarm system cameras. He was exhausted.

As we were learning more about mental health with our daughters and how we could best help them, our psychologist aided us to see that Ken was struggling with his own. Over thirty years of managing inmates and offenders had taken its toll. There were too many files Ken had read that contained too much information about the horrific acts' humans were capable of. There were too many inmates and offenders who continued to try and deceive Ken and the system. Just too much negativity all welling up from Ken's desire to help people whose actions had landed them on the wrong side of the law. The gang attack on our home took all those years of caustic bombardment and wrapped it up into an intolerable condition called PTSD – Post Traumatic Stress Syndrome.

Post-Traumatic Stress Syndrome is a term often associated with soldiers who have witnessed the horrors of war, police officers, victims of abuse and now Ken. PTSD is a mental health condition triggered by a terrifying event or culmination of events. Ken needed a break. He needed to find some goodness in the world again and let some sunshine into his heart. We found support from our psychologist, who couldn't believe what had happened just after we met her.

She turned out to be a much needed lifeline for us. Ken needed to take a step back, take care of himself for a while. There was just too much! We pulled back from so many things. It was almost like receding into a little cave so we could take care of our wounds. A favourite quote of mine is from the Stars Wars Movies. Yoda says to Luke Skywalker, "Do or do not, there is no try." I disagree. There is only try. Try and try and try again. Keep going, never give up and give yourself time to try again.

We needed time. We pulled back from completing anymore podcasts. It took too much energy and we both needed to find our smiles again.

How could we inspire a message of hope for others when we ourselves were grasping at the rope thrown down the well of our despair?

In the midst of all this mayhem, my insurance company decided that since I had been away from work for so long, they needed proof that I couldn't work. The notes from both my family doctor and the neurologist weren't enough. I think part of it is standard protocol, but our cups were very full, and anything extra caused the vitriol we were living in, to spillover. I had to go to a specialized clinic for a "Functional Capacity Assessment".

I was nervous and couldn't shake the feelings of guilt. This appointment, my problem, was adding to our full deck of stress. At the clinic I first had an interview. As the assessor looked at my doctor's notes and asked many questions, he wondered out loud why we were there. He said he had never had a stroke survivor need to complete this "Functional Capacity Assessment". We agreed but they were being paid to do it, so we started. Many of the tasks enhanced my overall dizziness. By lunchtime I wasn't feeling very good, and I could tell my anxiety was increasing.

They needed to take my blood pressure, as per my doctor's note. I was still living with the risk of another bleed. The stress of the appointment and the tasks had my blood pressure increasing. The staff had no idea what to do. They had never encountered a situation like this. Ken knew what to do. He called my doctor and explained the circumstances. She immediately ordered that they stop all assessments.

I was overwhelmed and started crying. This was just too much. We returned home, feeling defeated. Home wasn't even our refuge anymore, where we felt safe and protected. The next day the insurance company called and said even though I refused to complete the assessments they had enough information to grant me continued financial support. I told them I hadn't refused; I couldn't do it anymore. The agent just kept repeating that I refused. Ken took over the call and it ended politely enough, knowing that they would continue their support.

It was such an egregious position to be in. I wanted more than anything to be back at work. The doctors and my own brain and body prevented me from returning. Then insurance made me feel like I was trying to cheat them into supporting me. Their job is the one job I could never do, ever! The insurance agents must be a rare breed. Or maybe, life providing me with more insight and seeing what Ken had to deal with day after day at work, they had seen too many cases where people were cheating and had the wool pulled over their eyes too many times.

We were exhausted, from stress, from fear, from anxiety. With continued support from our psychologist Ken finally took time off work. Now he could concentrate on himself. Our youngest daughter was still struggling with her own mental health and our eldest daughter had sent an email, removing herself even further from our family. I was crushed and resorted to what I did best.

GOLD NUGGETS

I embraced denial. I locked all these problems into different boxes and stored them in my brain. Mostly it worked but every so often, one of the boxes opened a crack, usually in the middle of the night. My grief flowed out into the darkness, the night hiding my tears, keeping my secrets. I woke up exhausted but kept going. I thanked God for another day and promised to try and help others.

In helping others, I found relief from the constant pain of my own life. Between my concerns for my children, dealing with the loss of my career, still discovering what my new normal was and now, our own home not being safe, I needed those little bits of gold in all the mud of my existence.

One of the gold nuggets was a new endeavour we embarked on. I have always been an avid reader. When we lived in Grande Cache, I was on the library board. The best part was seeing all the new books and attending the annual Library Conference. The next best part was getting a first-hand look at all the newest children's books and sharing them with my own children. I loved kid's books and I volunteered to host a Saturday morning children's story time. I enjoyed picking out and reading the stories and I think the kids did too. One Saturday I was reading nursery rhymes and ended with the "Three Little Kittens" and had hidden mittens all over the library. A few were hidden too well, and the staff discovered mittens in odd places for several days.

Our house was always bursting with books for the kids. I loved reading to my children. I would make different voices and try to add dynamics whether it was scary, funny, or adventurous. Their favourite was a dramatic tale, called "Dogzilla", about a hairy pooch terrorizing the city of Mousetropolis! When we went on road trips, I bravely controlled the queasiness that reading created while being a passenger in a car. I read almost the entire Harry Potter series out loud to them. Reading and writing has always been my passion and I have written a few children's books just for our family.

One was inspired by my mom. At home, growing up, she would always tell us, "Close the fridge door before the penguins come" as my sisters or I would stare into the refrigerator, deciding on a snack. I wrote a whole kids' story about it, complete with penguins appearing in the kitchen. My own children loved the story and were as familiar with the phrase as I was.

Another time, my sister was coming for a visit with her two young children. Her youngest was terrified of dogs and we had one big, hairy dog at the time. He was as friendly and lovable as they come but how do you convince a young child who is afraid? My answer was to write a book. It was a story of my niece meeting our big, furry beast. My sister illustrated it. The book achieved its goal, and my niece and our dog became good friends. She now has a big, hairy dog of her own.

My newest gold nugget was also my newest mission; to try and help children. I wanted to write a children's book about stroke. The inception for the idea first came when we were doing a podcast with a dear family friend. He had been a friend of our eldest daughter and now he was working hard to complete his doctorate in neuroscience. He was interested in everything brainy and helped us out by being a guest.

While we were chatting after the recording was done, he had coined the term, Ty the Neuro Guy. Immediately ideas flooded into my head. Why not create a superhero dedicated to helping children learn about stroke and the brain. It was an exciting idea. Maybe there was an element of my own regret of not having sought professional support for my children after my stroke.

When I shared my thoughts with Ken, he loved it. Ken always fully supports my ideas and helps me bring them to fruition. I got to work on the book. The words came quickly, refining them took a lot more effort. I had some definitive ideas on how I wanted to present stroke.

First was to name our superhero. Ty was already a superhero. We needed one just for our books. I did some research. After a few failed attempts at things like Cerebral Sally and Brainy Bob I came up with Glia Girl. Glial cells are cells in our brains that help the neurons do their job better. They are very helpful cells and the perfect name for the superhero helping kids learn about brains.

I wanted the superhero to be a girl. I feel girls need more role models of females doing amazing things. I was part of that focus group for women in non-traditional roles when I worked at the steel mill. I didn't want Glia Girl to be a typical female, with curves and beautiful hair. Instead, I envisioned her as a lumpy, bumpy, brainy bodied being. Our gender shouldn't be tied to how we look.

I felt I had a great tale aiding kids to understand what a stroke is. I also wanted to make stroke less scary while empowering kids by letting them know they can help too. I wanted it to be filled with hope and lessen the feelings of doom when you hear the diagnosis of stroke. I also wanted the person who had a stroke to be an Auntie instead of Grandma. I'm living proof that stroke can strike at any age! Now the challenge was finding someone to illustrate it.

A children's book needs to have pictures. Vibrant, fun illustrations breathe life into the words and keep children engaged in the story. I had asked a few people with no success when again, the universe intervened and made available what we needed. My sister had told me, and I believe it to be true, tell the universe what you want and when you are ready it will come. It's also called prayer.

We were ready. Kevin had worked with an arts teacher at his school. This wonderful, talented teacher had previously illustrated another children's book. As fate would have it, they were casually talking at work when her past experience and my stroke came up. Almost magically, her talent met my need. Kevin introduced us virtually. It was the start of a beautiful collaboration.

This kind and gifted illustrator brought my words to life. She took my vision and put a face to it. Glia Girl became real through her brush strokes and water colours. The two main children developed faces and smiles. It was a year and a half of seeing the pictures being created and then putting them together with my words.

Then came the nitty gritty work. To save costs, we formatted the book ourselves. Self-publishing is not cheap. Luckily, the publishing company offered lots of free advice on how we could do it ourselves and what we needed to do so they could print it without additional costs. I became an expert on resizing, rewriting and Microsoft Publisher.

The biggest challenge was in the story itself. Less is more and I had too many words per page. I needed to shrink the number of words I used without changing the essence of my story. Rewrite after rewrite, and multiple formatting attempts, it was a slow work in progress. Between waiting for the amazing illustrations to be completed and then properly formatting and rewriting, it took me well over a year to finish it.

TWITTER & COVENANT HEALTH

We needed something bright in our lives to look forward to and the book was only one small part. I still needed to be busy to keep all those boxes in my brain under lock and key. I became familiar with Twitter and started posting daily. Surprisingly, I found a supportive online group of fellow stroke and traumatic brain injury (TBI) survivors. Their posts gave me inspiration and understanding.

Their honest quotes on the challenges of surviving a stroke or TBI blew fresh air into my clouded thoughts of how I felt my recovery should be going. With these posts I was able to be gentler with myself, and more compassionate. Slowly, I was taking more steps towards acceptance. Then another opportunity came to me as well. Again, just at the right time.

A month before Christmas I was asked to join a volunteer council, as a patient advisor. This was something I had never heard of, but it piqued my interest. It was with Covenant Health, the Catholic branch to Alberta Health Services. The council was officially called "Patient, Resident and Family Advisory Council" or PRFAC. It was a combination of staff and volunteers. All the volunteers had some type of "lived experience" with healthcare.

Our council was tasked with offering our own personal stories, feedback, and advice to Covenant Health and their different departments to assist with helping every patient, resident, and their families to have the best healthcare experience possible, despite the outcome. It was a dream to be offered a spot on the council. It was a way I could give back, help others, and keep my brain busy. I was so honoured to be a part of it since its inception with Covenant Health. I still am.

The first meeting was just before Christmas. Again, I was thankful for something else to focus my attention on. Christmas was a tough one that year, on many levels. Our eldest daughter was still estranged and for the first time since she was born, we would go through Christmas without one word from her. The presents under the tree for her and her wife were left unclaimed.

But the most outrageous and difficult were the presents under the tree from Ken's Mom and Dad. Very unexpectedly, Ken's mom passed away, just before Christmas. Ken had been talking to her just days before. She had ongoing health issues, but she seemed fine on the phone, full of good spirits and her usually natty humour. It was unbelievable and we were stunned.

One morning, at the house she shared with Ken's dad, her husband of 61 years, she just didn't wake up. Didn't things like this only happen in the movies? Bad movies? It was beyond mind blowing. I had known her since I was a teenager. I couldn't comprehend how Ken must have been feeling.

To say it was a difficult time would be an understatement. Ken was still trying to manage his own mental health hardships from the gang attack on our house. And we had presents under the tree from Ken's mom, but we no longer had her, only all our heart-felt memories. She had gotten them for us before she passed. It would be two years until we were able to give our eldest daughter the ones for her; and then through someone else, not even during a happy reunion. Ours was the complete opposite of any of the seasonal Hallmark Christmas specials.

Our family came together, as best as we could, to support one another. We found succor in our shared grief. Our son, Kevin, suggested we all have a toast of Crown Royal, Gramma Jackson's favourite, in honour of her memory. Coming together, sharing memories, talking openly – those were the best balms to help manage the pain of the loss of someone we loved. Going forward though, time would be the best healer and just like my stroke, just like the gang attack, we would take it one day at a time.

Fortunately, my parents came and spent Christmas with us. Their love and support helped us to manage all the madness and find some Christmas spirit. We sang Christmas carols and carried out our Christmas traditions. All too soon the season was over, my parents returned home as did Kevin.

Without the love, support, and distraction those acerbic thoughts and feelings returned. It was just too much. Sometimes I felt like I was going to explode from the intensity and immensity of it. Before my stroke I used to go for a run, blasting my music to release the stored energy that would otherwise certainly do me in. Without that tool I had to look for other ways.

A favourite movie of mine, The Matrix, had the computer agent telling the hero that they tried creating a world where everyone was happy and did not experience any suffering. The agent said it was a disaster, no one was happy when they had everything they needed. Maybe we need hardships in our life to keep us motivated, to quell our competitive nature. Maybe without difficulty we can't appreciate all the good we have in our life. I know I took a lot of things for granted before my stroke. Always having my family around was the biggest.

Maybe humans need something to fight for, work towards, something that pushes us in a direction we wouldn't otherwise consider. Perhaps that is why these reality television shows are so popular. We can watch people facing unbelievable challenges and succeed or fail as they try to beat the odds. Maybe we just need reasons to take chances, feel that adrenaline, experience the natural high of our triumph.

At that moment I would have given anything for a world without hardships. I was living in the worst reality show, and I no longer wanted to be the star. I had to search for some other ways to release my powder keg of destructive emotions. I tried and was able to go on the treadmill. It wasn't quite the same but effective. I was able to go faster than in the outside world, being able to hold on and focus just on one spot, negating my symptoms. But what works, to some extent, and something I've used profusely in the last few years, is writing.

*"All journeys have secret destinations of which the
traveller is unaware." Martin Buber*

CHAPTER 3

WRITING AND DREAMS

Writing, taking those thoughts and feelings, letting them run through my brain, into my hand, and onto paper. It's almost as good as running and in some ways better. I have a permanent document of how I was feeling.

Some of those thoughts are pretty dark and when rereading I surprise myself with the depth of my feelings. But it was real at that moment. And it's both an ending and a beginning. Writing it down releases those negative feelings that were clutching my brain, holding me prisoner of my own thoughts. It provides an end to those thoughts. They are written down, a key to unlock my cell. I am able to walk out of my nefarious jail and start again. Those dismal thoughts are now written down, out of my head and there is room for new, more positive thoughts, a pathway of hope towards something lighter and brighter.

Even with writing, the stress was getting to me in ways I didn't realize. I started having bad dreams. Most of the dreams I didn't remember, although Ken sure did. I would rouse him from his own slumber, screaming at some unknown terror. They always left me with a feeling of dread. Ken was there for me, holding me until the dread subsided and I could again fall back asleep.

The most bothersome was a waking nightmare I had. Ken and I were driving one late afternoon. We had had a beautiful day in the country and were on our way home. I was sleepy but not sleeping. Suddenly, I was sure there was a car in our lane; headed right for us. We were on a crash course for a head on collision. I was sure we were going to die. I started screaming. Poor Ken, he grabbed me and started yelling "What, WHAT!" I looked ahead and there was no vehicle in our lane driving towards us. I started shaking, crying, and told Ken what I thought I had seen.

How Ken kept the car on the road through that, I'll never know. And he was able to comfort me, telling me it was okay, it was just a dream. But it wasn't! Was it? I was sure I was awake. It was all so confusing. Not long after, I had a night full of dreams that I will never forget. I wrote it down on the advice of both our psychologist and my sister. Here's what I wrote to recount that night of three dreams.

Throughout history, things have been said to come in threes. Bad luck, sneezes, the Holy Trinity. It is believed if an unfortunate incident has already occurred twice, it will most likely happen a third time. There are many examples of "the rule of three", in writing, economics, even aviation. I could go on and on but here is the story of the three that happened to me, ending with my wrists wrapped.

The Night of Three

I awoke to my husband, Ken, gently pushing on my shoulder, asking, "Are you okay?"

My head was fuzzy with remnants of a dream not quite remembered. He asked again, "Are you okay, you were moaning." I couldn't quite recall what had caused me to cry out in my sleep. I had a feeling of something dark and nebulous but without any substance of what it was. I was groggy with sleep accompanied by the ever-constant drunk dizziness I've had since my first stroke almost 3 years ago. Once Ken felt I was okay we both drifted back to sleep.

I begged her to tell me what had happened, to say something to me, her mother. My eyes beseechingly asking for some explanation for her abrupt

Christine Holubec-Jackson

departure from our lives. She absently shrugged her shoulders and proceeded to tell me that her life was better now. Life was easier and less stressful. She delivered this devasting news with a careless attitude, akin to someone declaring they now only take one lump of sugar in their tea instead of two.

I crumbled inside. I implored her to let me be part of her life, to tell me what I had done wrong, give me a chance to fix it. She rolled her eyes and glanced towards another person. Not thinking it possible, I crumbled even more, torn apart, my sobs welling up from the bottomless fount of my despair.

"Are you okay?" Hands roughly shook my arm. My consciousness slowly returned as the dream started to loosen its iron grip on my mind. I had again awoken my husband with my nocturnal distress. The dream was so real and the feelings it invoked so profound I couldn't bear to repeat it. I told Ken I was okay and sorry for waking him. He tenderly stroked my arm, telling me it was all okay. Holding hands, we both fell back asleep.

The house was new to me but held some familiarity I couldn't identify. My youngest daughter Emily was there as well as two other young women, whom I knew, yet didn't. We chatted amiably but I don't know what about. Underlying it was a feeling that something needed to be taken care of. I was the eldest, the mother-figure, I should take care of it.

I was in another room. I could hear the girls chatting. The door was partially open. I looked up and there on the wall was a figurine. It's head, shoulders and hands were made of wood, the rest a rough knitted material. It looked like a type of circus jester from the distant past. It was wearing a funny hat, had a pointed nose, make-up to accentuate the nose and lips. Its cheeks were two red circles.

It started talking to me. It should have been surprising but somehow, I expected it. This was the reason I had appeared in this room. I can't say "came" to the room as I had no idea how I got there. I looked up at the figurine and without real words we both knew I was there to settle the score, take care of the problem. The figurine was still attached to the wall and tried to convince me that the stuffed animal on the floor behind me was what I had come for, that it was the real problem.

I looked at the stuffy. It was grey and pink, laying face down. I couldn't quite tell what it was, but I guessed it could be an elephant. I looked back at the figurine, knowing It was the problem. I would not be fooled. Then suddenly, it came to me. A solution so simple, to take the evil away, to fix the problem. I had to sand the wooden parts of the figurine. By sanding It, I would literally rub away the wickedness. Our lives could become filled with sunshine and goodness again.

I tugged the figurine off the wall. I held It down in front of me and foolishly told It what I was planning. I thought maybe some part of It wanted to be rid of the malevolence within. The painted face turned sinister. The rough knitted parts suddenly grew and snaked around my wrists. My hands were bound but I refused to give up. I started running to where Emily and the other girls were, the figurine becoming part of me as it bound my wrists tighter. I cried out, "Help" three times.

For the third time, Ken shook my arm. "Christine, Christine…. Are you okay? What's going on?" I woke up, disorientated. Figments of my dream mixed with reality. "You were crying out, what happened?" queried Ken. I told him about the evil figurine and how it tied my wrists. Ken was concerned. So was I.

The dream had been so real. Ken comforted me and soon the dream started to recede, a little. It had been so vibrant, in colours, details, feelings. It would take some time for this one to truly fade. I managed a little more sleep. When I got up in the morning, it was still dark, as it is in winter in Alberta. I had some trepidation as I went downstairs to make my tea. All was calm and quiet in our house. I sipped my tea and found some comfort. Over the next several days I mused over the dream, trying to find some meaning.

Sometimes a dream is just that, a dream. Reading too much into it or trying to find meaning can be a wasted endeavour. But sometimes there is a message. The trick is trying to ascertain which is which. Maybe analysis and interpretation will put these dreams to bed (pun intended). Maybe I was trying to lock the memory into the computer screen on which I typed them, in my desire to understand.

I think my dreams of three were significant, filled with messages. I don't believe they were portents of things to come but rather a look into my subconscious. My dreams delved into what I'm trying to keep under lock and key during the daytime hours.

My first dream I have no conscious memory of so there's nothing to analyze except it was something that bothered me enough to wake Ken. Maybe it was a precursor of what was coming.

My second dream is one of my greatest fears. Aside from some type of grievous harm coming to any of my children my greatest fear has become reality with my first-born child. She has removed herself from me, from her entire immediate family. The connection between truth and fantasy is not hard to make with this dream.

The third dream is ripe with many meanings and interpretations. In letting my thoughts run free to roam around the inner recesses of my brain, perhaps are some of the subconscious feelings let loose.

- The figurine represents the darkness in my life created by a multitude of events.
    - ◊ My stroke.
    - ◊ My eldest's elopement and estrangement.
    - ◊ My youngest daughter's struggles with mental health.
    - ◊ The gang attack on our house, targeting Ken.
    - ◊ The unexpected death of Ken's mother.
- The deflection from the figurine towards the stuffy represents the senselessness of it all as well as my daughter's last message to me listing some benign reasons for her estrangement.
    - ◊ The stuffy being face down may also represent my feeling of being in the dark, not knowing the true reasons behind the alienation. Or it could be, more literal, in that she has turned her back on us, or I have turned my back on facing my feelings.
- Even in my dream, I tried to focus on the problem, the figurine, coming up with a solution; sanding It would erase the evil and the wickedness It brought into the world.

- When my wrists were bound by the figurine, my helplessness in not being able to fix the problems in my life were highlighted.
- I realized I needed help and ran to get it. If Ken had not woken me up would a solution have revealed itself? I don't think so as there is no easy answer, no quick fix. My fear was real and transpired from dream to consciousness when I called out for help. Ken was there for me.

Nothing has changed because of my dreams except knowing I needed to find some tools to cope with what was happening in my life. I kept it locked in a box and tried to maintain my façade that life was good. I tried to help others and I tried to keep busy. Behind all my busyness was this hole in my heart that couldn't be filled and was bubbling over into my dreams. It wasn't the first of crying out in my sleep and it wouldn't be the last. I've had more bad dreams, have woken Ken up but nothing compared to that one night of three bad dreams.

A Chinese proverb says, "Fortune does not come twice. Misfortune does not come alone.", meaning good things only come once while bad things will always come in groups. Do I believe this, I'm not sure? We've had more than our share of bad, but we've also had more than one good thing. I am grateful. And I am more than grateful to be able to put pen to paper to relieve some of my apprehension.

And just when the dreams had faded into something not so significant, the poignant edges softened by time, I had 3 eggs, from my regular carton of 12 large eggs, with double yolks. Mmmmmmh.

Bad dreams notwithstanding, life continued, and we tried to find positive things to focus on. The egg yolks meant nothing, and I tried not to see portents of evil in every situation.

"Life brings a lot of noise; you gotta focus on what really matters." Anonymous

CHAPTER 4

COVID & CONTROL

The house was too quiet, even though Emily had moved back home in the fall. So, I focused my energy on continuing the Glia Girl book and my volunteer work with Covenant Health. But to quote my mom now, "nothing ever gets so bad it can't get worse", the world entered a pandemic. Yes, just as we were seeing the finish line of our book, COVID-19 struck. Well, if we didn't have bad luck, we wouldn't have any at all, or so the saying goes.

COVID-19 brought unprecedented times for the entire world. We all banded together, to make the best of it. Kevin and his wife, Alix, had to learn how to teach students online. Emily, with one and half years left of university also moved to online learning. We entered the time of Zoom calls, online meetings, masks and disinfecting our groceries. We diligently watched the daily updates and saw the numbers of infections climb.

Everyone thought it would be several weeks and life would resume its usual, in-person hectic lifestyle. COVID-19 had a different plan. We developed a new routine, including praising the heroic work of healthcare workers and all essential workers. There was a feeling of "we're all in this together!"

The pandemic dragged on. It affected everyone a little differently and Emily, our youngest, still struggled with mental health. Her doctor had suggested that getting a big dog might be a good idea. Ken jumped on board with the idea. With his continued apprehension of a possible home invasion, he wanted a big dog. The dog would fulfill three purposes, his big bark could scare away potential invaders, his size could offer protection and it was just what the doctor ordered for Emily's mental health.

The only one skeptical about this idea was me. We still had our gentle, cuddly Twinkie. An elderly Shi Tzu who was my couch buddy. She had been faithfully by my side since my first stroke. Her ageing and not being able to walk as far helped us to discover another benefit.

Since my second small brain bleed, I always used a walking pole when I went out. Balance was still an issue as was dizziness. It was a beautiful spring that year and with COVID-19, Ken and I were going on more walks together. As my endurance increased, we were limited on our walks by how far Twinkie could make it. She was nearly sixteen years old and long walks were no longer an option.

Ken, always the problem solver, researched and found a dog stroller perfect for Twinkie. It would be my Mother's Day present. It was perfect and a perfect distraction. I wasn't looking forward to Mother's Day very much. My grasp of my own motherhood felt tenebrous. Any compliments delivered my way seemed dishonest. My heart was broken, I didn't know how to fix it and I didn't know how to help my daughters.

Before my first stroke, I often was the organizer of our family. I kept things together, planned and dealt with many of the small problems. It wasn't that Ken didn't do it; he fulfilled his parental jobs in other ways. We each had our roles and it seemed to work. Suddenly, I couldn't do it anymore. Stroke had changed me. Ken's time was spent worrying about me, not about the roles I could no longer do. We were just happy I was still alive. We didn't have the capacity to see the all-encompassing, life altering effects of stroke at that time.

We had watched several television programs that seemed to deliver a message just for us. It was about families who had been torn apart by divorce, a death or some other life-altering event to one of the parents. Maybe these shows were reminding us that what we were going through was tough and not to expect such an incident to leave us unscathed.

But I never imagined that three years, post-stroke, we would still be dealing with acceptance. I am a slow learner, but perhaps acceptance of who you are is a lifelong commitment. We all go through events and experiences that change who we are. Some are smaller, like a freak hailstorm destroying your trees and punching holes in the siding of your house[2] and some are mind-blowing, life altering, like having and surviving a stroke. But each result in some type of change. How we respond to these life experiences adds layers to our character, to who we are.

On that thought, on the one year anniversary of the gang attack on our house, our friend and neighbour died. One neighbour suspected he might be in distress, so we banded together with other neighbours and the RCMP to break down his door. We found him deceased in his own home. He was the same age as Ken.

We were there to support his family, but we never did find out what caused his sudden and unexpected death. We guessed that maybe it was undiagnosed COVID-19, but we'll never know for sure. The neighbourhood was saddened by his sudden, unexpected death but it was the height of COVID-19 so there was no funeral or celebration of life to provide any solace. It was another Stygian life experience.

Ken and I appreciated again our life together and that we were alive! Even though I felt like the Cruella de Vil of mothers, I celebrated life, and the fact Twinkie needed me. With the stroller we found something that would improve both our lives. Twinkie was a little nervous but soon appreciated the view and the rest. She would sit up and look around, even bark at other dogs. She was a funny doggie though. She knew when we turned around to go back home. At that point she wanted out of the stroller. In her little dog brain, she thought we would get home faster if she walked herself.

An unexpected benefit ensued. With the support of the stroller, my own walking improved dramatically. I was more stable; my walking was more even. I didn't stumble or have any "drunk" looking movements. And I could walk faster. The dog stroller became what my one sister

---

2   In 2017, we had a devastating hailstorm that punched holes in the siding of our house and ruined all our gardens.

had been recommending since my first stroke: a walker! There was no stopping me now.

NEW DOG

Back to welcoming a new dog into our family. Things happened so fast. While I was thinking we were in the discussion phase of welcoming a new pet, Ken and Emily were buying supplies. Before I knew it, Ken and I were driving out to a farm to pick up Emily's new puppy. (Emily had been called in to work and couldn't go herself) How did this happen? My anxiety skyrocketed and I was filled with trepidation over this new addition.

But then Arthur stole my heart. That's the name Emily bestowed on the Chesapeake Bay Retriever, Chocolate Labrador Cross puppy. He was adorable. We had met his mother and grandmother at the farm, and they were smaller labs, maybe sixty pounds. That relieved some of my anxiety over getting a big dog. (Arthur grew to be around ninety pounds! He certainly didn't take after his mama.)

It's remarkable how situations thrust upon you can change your mind. I had never wanted a Labrador Retriever of any kind, but especially not a chocolate one. I can offer no good reason why. I never wanted a big dog again. We had one when we lived in the mountains, a perfect place for a big dog, and it was still a lot of work. And I really didn't want a dog that shed. No way!

Arthur punched through every preconceived prejudice I had about big, hairy, chocolate lab crosses. Although he was technically Emily's dog, with her living at home, he became the family dog. She was still busy with her last year of university and managing her challenges with mental health. Arthur brought a lot of laughter into our house. He was the bright spot in our lives, chasing away the darkness brought on by strokes, gang attacks, mental health and now COVID-19.

Twinkie wasn't too impressed with the addition, but Arthur loved her unconditionally. He even wanted to be in the stroller with her when we went for walks. Twinkie put up with his antics and when she had enough, found a quiet spot to rest. Sadly, shortly after Arthur came, Twinkie was diagnosed with an aggressive form of cancer and soon crossed the Rainbow Bridge. We will always miss her, and her quiet, cuddly demeanor.

It's funny how things always seem to happen all at once. We were just settling into having Arthur in our house when our hot water tank blew, flooding our basement. Due to COVID-19, it was challenging to get someone in to replace the tank. Our flooded basement caused a lot of extra work and in the midst of it is when we had to say good-bye to Twinkie. Time stopped for a moment. Then ramped right back up with the enormity of fixing our basement.

Arthur provided a much needed balm for all that was happening. He seemed to sense what was going on and was extra snuggly instead of his usual puppy antics. He needed us and needed care, taking our minds off everything else and helping us to manage the grief of losing Twinkie.

Going for walks was very different. The stroller was such a benefit to my walking, I continued using it when we took Arthur out. Occasionally he would want to sit in it, not because he was tired but for the novelty of it. It never lasted long and soon he was wriggling with energy that the stroller could not contain. My sister, Cami, tried not to say I told you so about the benefits of a walker, but she did tell me so and she was right.

Although Arthur was Emily's dog, I loved taking him for walks. Soon I was going every day, sometimes even twice a day. He had an endless supply of energy. Emily introduced us to a term we had not heard of but with Arthur it soon became common. He often experienced the "zoomies". He would race with uncontrolled energy in circles around the backyard. He would jump as he ran by, hoping to get the mitt I still wore on my left hand.

Emily enrolled him in puppy training classes to manage his growing size and energetic behaviour. Usually, I or Ken would go with her and then with her busy class schedule, just Ken and I took Arthur. That's when we discovered how shy he was. If the instructor came to talk to him, he immediately piddled and hid behind one of us. Slowly, slowly, Arthur came out of his shell, but he was a COVID-19 dog. He had very little contact with other people. The effects of COVID-19 were far reaching, and in the most unexpected ways.

One of the positive disruptors (a term I learned through my volunteer work with Covenant Health) was breaking down barriers to connecting with others. Everyone got creative in connecting now that the world was living in mandatory isolation. Using virtual tools such as Zoom, Microsoft Teams and What's App skyrocketed. For me, as much as I missed face-to-face contact, there were some real benefits.

The PRFAC volunteer advisory council I was a part of turned to Zoom meetings. We had had only two in-person meetings when COVID-19 hit. I could drive but since the last small bleed, highway driving was challenging. With virtual meetings Ken didn't need to schedule time off to take me to my quarterly meetings. We had shorter meetings via Zoom. It wasn't as big a deal for me to participate. Before, I had to plan the day before and day of to manage attending a meeting. My energy levels were still fragile and looking around at all the different faces took effort.

Some of the other things I participated in were now on hold, so I found myself with more time. I was able to concentrate on my Twitter posts and monthly newsletters. I appreciated the community I was developing through Twitter. I know many people complain about Twitter, but I found a group of like-minded people. Many were stroke survivors but there were others who wanted to spread messages of hope, faith, compassion, inspiration, kindness, and fun.

I discovered someone in the southern USA whose love of oatmeal surpassed my own, @101Fix. Her creativity of oatmeal recipes was as vast as the thought provoking quotes, she included. I connected with another stroke survivor in Ireland. His tweets really helped me to allow some compassion for myself and what it meant to be a stroke survivor. I tried to post inspiration and information, but I gained so much more than what I tweeted.

Years post-stroke don't matter. Stroke is a life-long change. Reading other survivors posts, or Thrivers, as @ThrivePlayer in Ireland called it, I learned so much. Many people go through life-altering events but reading all these various posts got me to thinking. People who have survived stroke or any type of brain injury, whatever the cause are different. Other diseases can be calamity causing but a brain injury changes the fundamental core of your being.

Reading multiple posts about this broke through the clouds and let in a beam of sun that highlighted why brain injury is so different. It aided me in making progress in my continuous journey of acceptance. Other survivors were still discovering their new normal, many years post stroke or other types of brain injury. It may seem excessive but to me it made a certain kind of sense. My belief is we possess an innate sense of who we are, from the moment we are born. As we go through life, experiences shape how we grow and develop. But that fundamental core, the part that makes me – me and you – you, is still there, no matter the layers that life adds.

RAMBLING AND THE SKY

Challenges, opportunities, the good and the bad, we respond to from the underlying essence of who we are. When something happens that changes your brain, whether a stroke or a traumatic brain injury or whatever, it causes a shift in your core. The crux of your being has been altered. Your new normal is aware of your past essence but it can no longer quite grasp what it really was. You've lost that nucleus that made you, you. It wreaks havoc within you because that sixth sense is desperately trying to find what has been lost.

I know I am rambling here but I'm still trying to grasp the changes within me. Many people, even today, compliment me on how well I am doing and that it seems there is nothing wrong with me. They say I look totally normal. Thank you very much but there is a private war going on inside. Not only am I managing the physical challenges of stroke, but I am still searching for the lost part of what made me, me. It's an ongoing battle. Most of the time, it is okay, I AM managing and grateful for where I am and what I have. But that sixth sense or whatever you want to call it knows part of me is gone and I can't stop trying to find it or replace it.

The best analogy I've thought of is that before brain injury I agreed with the rest of the world that the sky is blue. After my brain injury the sky is no longer the same, it is different, but I can't explain it to non-brain injury survivors what it is I am really seeing because they can only recognize that the sky is still blue. They may politely agree, but the true belief evaporates when they look up on a sun-shiny day and see a bright blue sky. That's the challenge in trying to describe the difference inside of you when you have an invisible injury. When someone with a brain injury looks at the sky, it isn't blue.

Connecting with others, through Twitter, via Zoom or other ways, really helped. Other stroke and brain injury survivors understood the "sky not blue" analogy. Despite COVID-19 and all the other challenges life had tossed our way, I was celebrating four years post stroke. I was busy with my children's book, volunteering with Covenant Health and managing our own family dynamics.

I kept busy, that's how I liked it. I couldn't leave too much room in my brain to ruminate. It seemed strange that my life could be described as hectic. I was only in my early fifties, retired and my recovery was still progressing; not the leaps and bounds I saw initially, but little milestones, mostly in finally accepting my new normal. I was only turning 53 at the end of April. My birthday and my stroke survival day are the same: four years ago, on my 49th birthday, I was in the special care unit of the hospital. Four years later, things seemed to be settling down for us somewhat. Four years! I was starting to accept my new normal.

Emily had almost finished university. She was graduating despite managing mental health challenges and a global pandemic. It was an admirable achievement, considering the personal mountain she was climbing. She had applied for and gotten a job in Jasper, the federal mountain park in western Alberta. She just wanted to get away for a while and have some adventures. We supported her in this dream, it would be good for her to have some adventure.

KEN'S SHOULDER

We were just starting to renovate our basement. Even though our band was still on a COVID-19 hiatus, we were confident we would get back to it soon. Ken had a vision of our basement as a perfect jam space. It was a Friday; Ken was done with work for the day. We were going to have an excellent evening, taking a break from renovations, and planning the release of our Glia Girl book, it was almost completely done. Emily was with a friend taking candid graduation photos around the university.

It was one of those moments. Time seemed to slow down, almost like the slo-mo setting on your phone. There should have been enough time to stop it, to save the day. There was enough time for a million thoughts to flit across my brain, flooding my thoughts.

Ken, just finished for the day, came upstairs and we were going to take Arthur for a walk. We still had a small gate to keep Arthur in the kitchen. As Ken stepped over, one leg snagged on the top. Ken stumbled a bit but caught himself. To recover, he quickly stomped the snagged leg down and pulled his other leg over. That's when it happened. Not quite balanced, the other foot fully got entangled in the two-foot-high moveable gate.

This is where the slo-mo comes in. As Ken was starting to crash, no hope of recovery, he looked at me, we locked eyes and time even stopped for a moment. We both knew he was going down. I tried to stop him, and he tried to twist, to soften the fall. Unfortunately, the wall was right there. He smashed his head and right shoulder into that darn wall. There's still a dent from where the side of his head hit, causing a minor concussion and ruining his glasses.

Ken sat up. I looked and immediately knew he had dislocated his shoulder. Ken then let out a loud string of colourful adjectives. His face turned ghostly white. We had to take him to the hospital. Several hours later, Ken was feeling much better. They had put his shoulder back in place and given him some effective pain medication. Recovery would be long; we had no idea how prolonged, or the hurdles life would insert along the way.

The next few weeks were tough. The emergency doctor had recommended Ken to see an orthopedic surgeon. The surgeon refused to take Ken on as a patient. No explanation, he just refused. Maybe this was fallout from the stresses of COVID-19. Ken saw his family doctor and had a referral to a different one. It would take seven months to see one and a lifetime of challenge awaited us in-between.

The doctor had recommended Ken take six weeks off work. I think Ken took about three. He didn't want to take much more; he had returned from his mental health leave after the gang attack several months earlier and felt bad for taking more time off. I was there to help as I could. We were used to Ken being the one who did the work when I was having a bad day. We had a role reversal. I started driving more, doing the shopping and took care of most of the cooking and cleaning.

I knew I was taking on too much but how could I not? Ken had been there for me for every step of the way throughout my entire stroke journey. It was time to give back and give him the comfort and care he deserved. Unfortunately, Emily left for Jasper shortly after the accident, so she was not able to provide much help.

Our gracious neighbours were ready and willing to help, offering to drive or help with yard work. As always, we tried to take care of business ourselves. After three weeks Ken decided he could go back to work. We did several trials of him driving. The actual driving was no problem but getting his seatbelt on and off created a challenge. When he first started back to work, several weeks later, I was there to help him but soon he figured out how to maneuver his right arm so his left arm could snap the belt into place.

What an ordeal. It was another prime example of how little control we actually have in our lives. As I always say, the only control we have is in how we respond to the loop de loops of life. We were doing the best we could and making the best of it. Ken disliked not being able to do what he wanted due to not being able to use his arm.

BASEMENT RENOS

The basement renovations were on hold, but we were so close. The next step was to finish painting. It would be much easier in our basement since there was no ceiling or floor to worry about marking with paint. Ken had done most of the patch work already, to fill various holes and dents.

This was something I could do. There were no ladders, no quick movements, just a little looking up. I could finish sanding and then paint the walls. I was thrilled to finally do something to help, to feel useful. Ken didn't feel right, sitting there while I worked. Now he got to experience how I felt when I was limited in my ability to help since my stroke.

The painting went quickly, quicker than I expected. I was enjoying doing some physical work again. My career at the steel mill had a physicality to it that I appreciated. Ken helped as much as he could and before we knew it, it was done. What next?

We took a weekend off, funny as neither of us were working at that time and went to visit Emily in Jasper. It was her twenty-second birthday, and she wasn't able to come home. Ken drove, with me helping with the seatbelt and changing gears.

It was a beautiful drive into the mountains and Arthur's first road trip. We were staying in the hotel where Emily had a housekeeping job. It was still COVID-19, but we had one vaccine already, so we felt a little better travelling. Jasper, usually a bustling tourist town, was more like a ghost town. It was only mid-May and COVID-19 lent its effect of isolation.

We loved it! To have this beautiful mountain town to ourselves. It was fabulous. We went on short hikes, Arthur got to go swimming and we could walk the streets with no crowds. I baked and brought a cake, and we ordered pizza for Emily's supper. The pizza was delivered so quickly and so hot, we had to let it cool enough to eat it. It seemed like the best pizza ever, gooey with just the right amount of saucy deliciousness.

I love being in the mountains. Ken and I lived thirteen years in the mountains, and I never stopped loving looking up at them every day. There is something so majestic about their colossal grand beauty; something humbling about being in the presence of something that that has been witness to time so ancient. My life is but a blip on the scale of time measured by these mountains. It's a good reminder to appreciate every moment we have. I was very grateful for our days immersed in the natural magnificence of the Rocky Mountains.

The weekend all too soon came to an end. Emily had discovered that housekeeping wasn't really her forte and had gotten another job, in that short stay we were there, on the Sky Tram. She would literally be working on top of a mountain, in the gift shop. Her commute would be on the gondola. It seemed like the perfect summer job. She was fulfilling her desire for some adventures.

Ken returned to work shortly after we returned. My time was still busier than usual, trying to do more at the house to ease the burden from Ken and his healing shoulder. He still was not able to lift his arm up in front or out to the side, at all. And there was still no appointment with an orthopedic specialist. He sought out a sport's physical therapist.

A clinic in Edmonton boasted experienced and knowledgeable therapists, specializing in bone, joint and muscle injuries. Ken went with hopes of regaining some movement in his right arm. The lack of improvement was cause for worry, but the therapist allayed his fears. He told Ken that an orthopedic specialist wouldn't be doing anything different and the only way to improve would be to do the exercises he prescribed and keep coming to the clinic.

Ken tried with no improvement whatsoever. We talked about these concerns and finally he went back to his family doctor to ask for further imaging to be done, just to check what kind of soft tissue damage may have occurred. Luckily this was faster than getting an orthopedic appointment. He was scheduled for an appointment for the beginning of July.

GLIA GIRL VIDEO

To help manage his lack of arm movement, I took on more of the household jobs. I was busier than ever with reflections of my previous, pre-stroke life peeking through my daily schedules. Within all this, we were also preparing to launch our Glia Girl children's book. We would do it virtually, thanks to COVID-19. I learned how to make an iMovie. I made a one-minute video, promoting Glia Girl and offering a competition. People who liked and shared the video on Twitter and Facebook would be entered into a draw to receive a free copy of our Glia Girl Book.

It was interesting learning how to make an iMovie, adding text and graphics. Kevin was there as my tech resource to help with my many questions. Once I was satisfied, I saved it, ready to release it in mid-June. The raffle for the books would be made June thirtieth. It was an exciting time and I felt things were moving in a positive direction. All this busyness had the added benefit of keeping my mind off Kaylyn and her continued separation from our family.

The unfinished basement was still gnawing away at Ken. He got in touch with one of Emily's friends to help. He was a very helpful and polite young man with an interest in history, especially the World Wars. They arranged a few days for him to come and help, between their work schedules. Emily was even able to come home for a few days to help. He was a very hard worker and a huge help to Ken. Initially, I took care of making meals and ensuring the coffee was hot.

After the second day, we realized I could do more. I became an essential part of the installation team. Ken was very limited in installing a ceiling, having the use of only one arm. Looking up is challenging for me, making me quite dizzy but I knew how much completing the basement meant to Ken. Between the four of us, we became two efficient teams.

I am adept at pushing myself, often to my own detriment. On the last day, I pushed, and I probably pushed too far. It was time to step back and rest. We ordered pizza for supper, and I let the others finish cleaning up. The job was done, we got through it. Ken with one arm and me with all my different impediments. Emily and her friend were essential, both with two working arms. There was a great feeling of accomplishment all around.

From all the hard work I knew I would need several down days to recover. I was slowly learning to live with the sword hanging over my head, and literally in my head. The abnormal blood vessel was still there, inoperable, but I felt I had reached a point where I was managing it and didn't let it take up too much time in my thoughts.

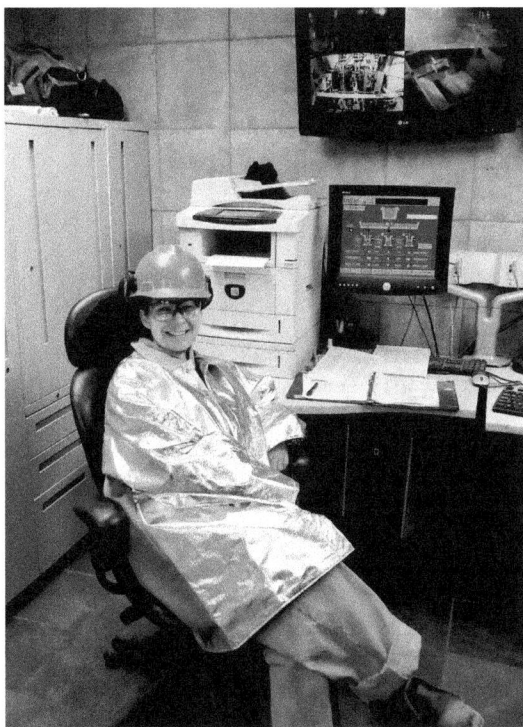

WORKING AT THE STEEL MILL.

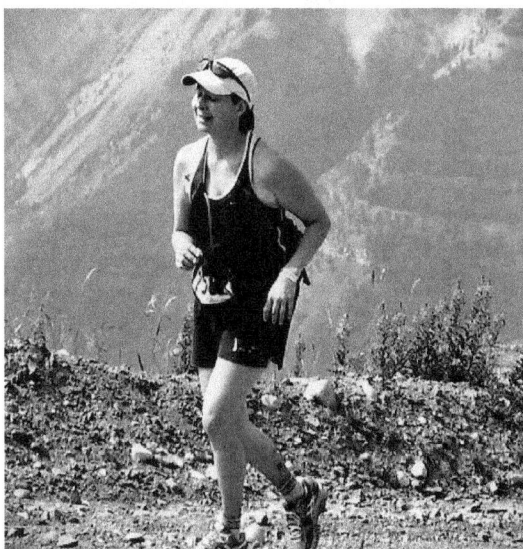

MY PRE-STROKE SELF, RUNNING A LEG OF THE CANADIAN DEATH RACE.

I Am Alive

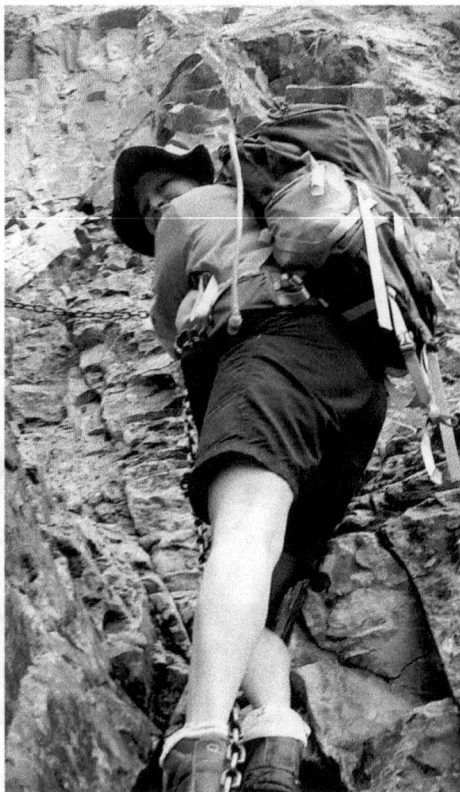

ENJOYING ONE OF MY PRE-STROKE ADVENTURES – BACKPACKING.

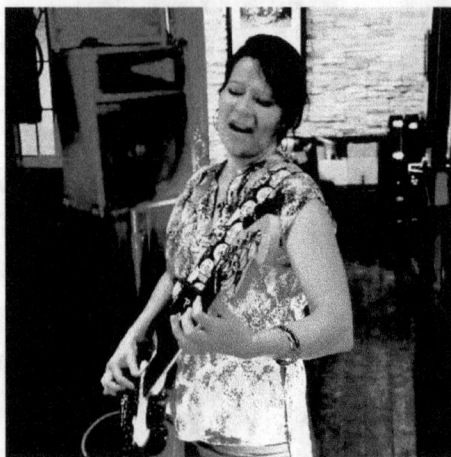

ME BASS PLAYING BEFORE STROKES. ALTHOUGH IT LOOKS MUCH DIFFERENT NOW, I'M SO THANKFUL I CAN STILL PLAY BASS.

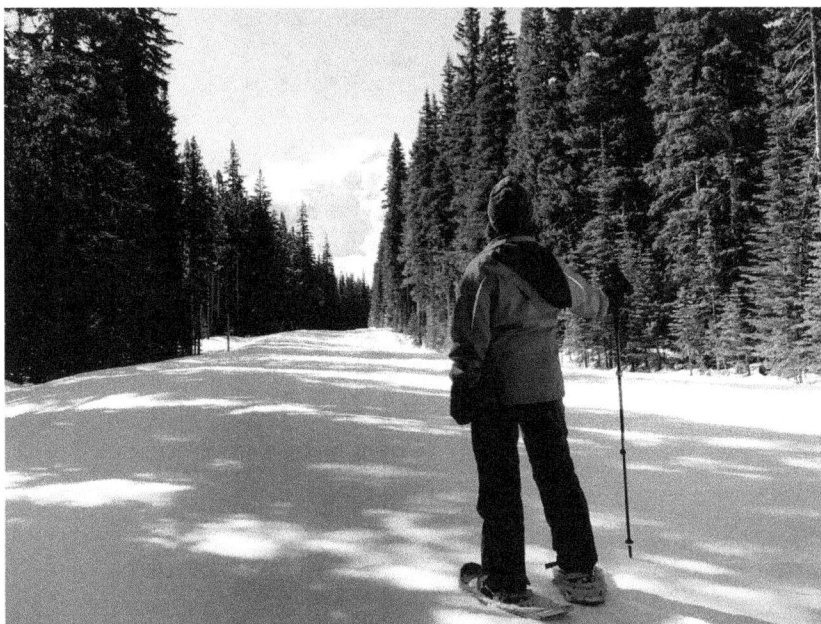

TWO WEEKS BEFORE MY FIRST STROKE I SNOWSHOED
14 KM'S UP AND DOWN A MOUNTAIN.

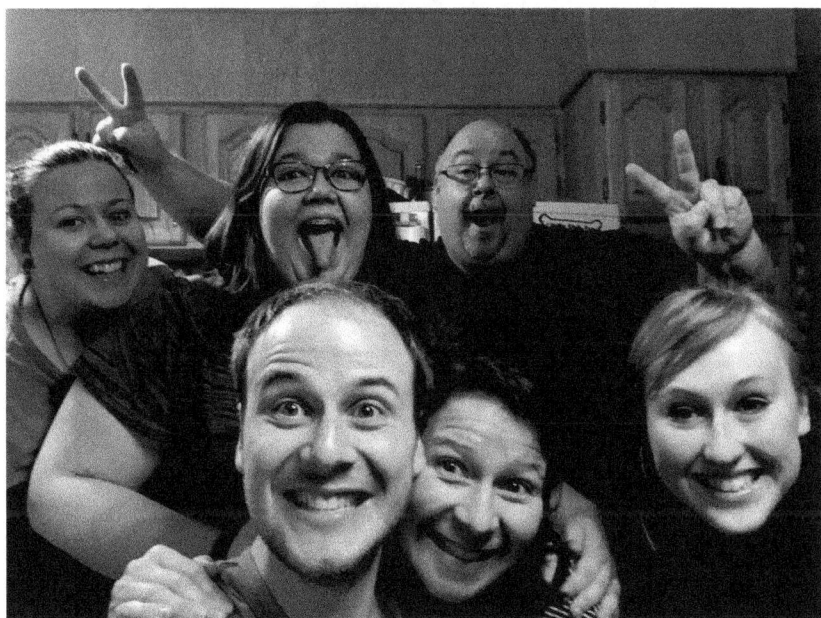

OUR HAPPY FAMILY! OH, TO HAVE THOSE MOMENTS AGAIN!

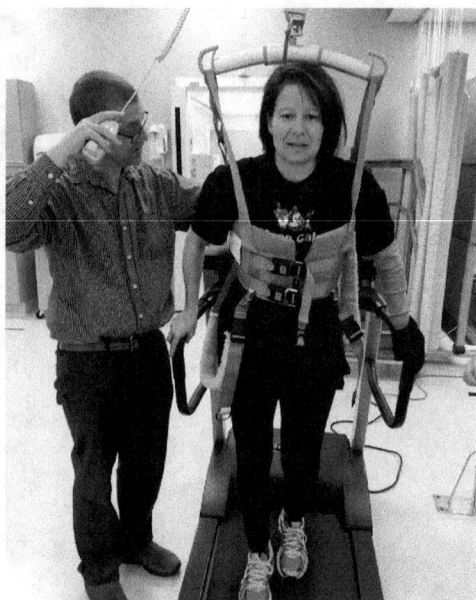

RECEIVING PHYSIOTHERAPY AFTER MY FIRST STROKE.
THERE WAS NO CHANCE OF ME FALLING!

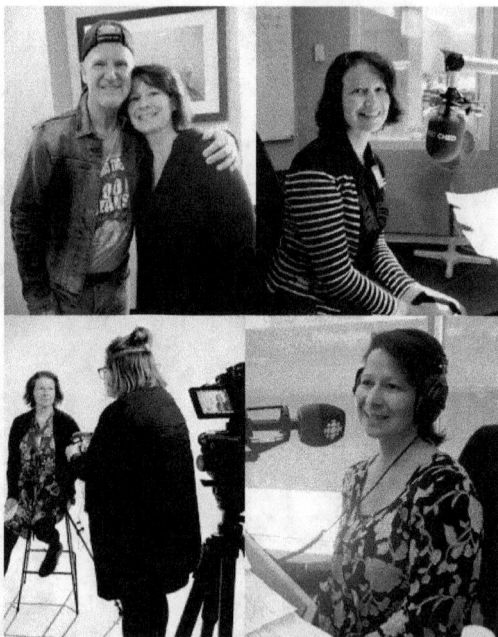

SHARING MY STORY – PODCASTS, RADIO AND COVENANT HEALTH.

Christine Holubec-Jackson

"The world breaks everyone and afterward many are stronger at the broken pieces." Ernest Hemingway.

CHAPTER 5

BLEEDING AGAIN

Soon, those ominous thoughts borne from the malformation in my brain were starting to creep back to the foreground. My recovery was slower than I expected. I was so tired and starting to feel dizzier. Our minds are amazing and the amount they try to protect us is incredible. Mine was doing just that. My old friend, Denial, was making a comeback, telling me a few more days of rest and I would be back to my new, old self.

A few days later I woke up feeling a little better, or so I thought. It was a bright, blue sky, sunny day. I had my usual cup of tea, did my Twitter post, and then took Arthur for our morning walk. I walked quite well with a pole but felt much sturdier when I had the running stroller to hold onto and push. Since Twinkie passed, Ken found a used running stroller that worked perfectly and even handled rougher trails. Using it, Arthur and I often walked up to three kilometers. People often looked forward to the baby they assumed was in my running stroller but there was no baby in mine. I just shook off any strange looks.

On that particular morning, as I went, the deep fatigue of post-stroke life started to settle into my bones, but there was something more to it. With every step, the ground was starting to undulate, as if I were walking on a wavy ocean, instead of a solid, paved path. When I looked ahead, the world was also moving, in contrast to my own movements.

Arthur was very well behaved; I think he could sense something was off. We turned around to go back home, much sooner than usual. Again, our amazing brains have an intuition, or perception that makes us aware, at an unconscious level, of a truth we are not yet ready to accept. I did not yet consciously grasp that anything could be wrong even though I knew it was. To me another brain bleed was incomprehensible. But at some level I knew, with some inexplicable certainty, that this would be the last walk Arthur and I would take together for a long time.

I am not totally irresponsible, and I have learned a lot since my first stroke. I was in so much denial with my first stroke that I still went to work while my brain was bleeding. I still drove home, a seventy-five-kilometer commute. I asked the neurologist when I could go back to work while he was telling me I had an inoperable, bleeding blood vessel in my brain stem.

No, I had learned. Even though it seemed inconceivable that anything bad was happening, I let Ken know how I was feeling, and I called my family doctor's office. Luck was with me, again. With my first stroke I had gotten a same day appointment with my amazing doctor. Ken made it for me while I was at work. Often it takes over two weeks to get in to see her. This time I was able to secure an appointment the next morning, over the telephone.

COVID-19 was still rampant, although vaccines were starting to make a difference. Ken and I had two by then and feeling like maybe an end to COVID-19 was in sight. The world was still learning how many things we could do virtually or just over the phone, hence the phone appointment. That subconscious intuitive part knew something was wrong, but I thought talking to my family doctor would make it better. My conscious, practical part just figured I was still recovering from the busyness of our basement work and extra duties around the house.

The next morning when I woke up, my subconscious intuition was starting to gain ground. My double vision was more pronounced, I lost the complete feeling of my left eye, and I was incredibly dizzy. I was glad about the morning phone appointment with my doctor, but I already knew she would instruct me to go to the neighbouring town to have a CT scan completed.

CT IN CAMROSE

In Alberta, not every hospital has the ability to manage strokes. Certain hospitals are given the designation along with the tools necessary to manage someone coming in presenting with stroke symptoms. We had learned so much while researching our podcasts. Our city, although the parameters for city in Alberta are small, was not a designated stroke hospital. Luckily, Camrose boasted a stroke unit and was only about a twenty-five-minute drive. I spent time there as a patient in the special care unit after my first stroke and that's where the Stroke, Early Supported Discharge program was based.

My doctor did not disappoint. On our phone call, I dug deep inside and without preamble, I told her I was worried I was having another bleed. I was surprised how difficult it was to say those words. A no nonsense, straight to the point person, she immediately told us to drive to Camrose, go to their emergency department and have a CT scan. She knew my history as well as my stubbornness, but I told her we would go right away. She had previously given Ken her personal cell phone number and asked him to text to keep her updated. Have I mentioned how incredible she is?

We arrived at the Camrose hospital and by this time, I knew something was definitely wrong. Despite that awareness, I still thought that it was just a small setback. I thought it would be like the other small bleed I'd had two years ago. I had managed, was okay, although with slightly more deficits. Familiarity breeds complacency, or maybe it was defiance, but I quelled my intuition and figured this was more of an inconvenience than a life-threatening emergency. I couldn't fathom the seriousness of my situation.

As always, the Camrose emergency department was filled with kind and compassionate staff. Very quickly I was sent off for a CT scan. A CT scan is computerized tomography that takes X-ray images of your body from different angles and uses computer processing to create cross-section images of bones, soft tissue and blood vessels. This would be my sixth.

The technician was very caring and even more so after my CT scan. From my understanding, when healthcare staff demonstrate excessive kindness, they are trying to soften the blow of bad news they know is coming. My worry increased but I still felt that this would just be a minor setback despite that inner voice whispering as softly as leaves rustling in a breeze, my true fears.

Back in the emergency room, Ken texted our family and let them know what was happening. Everyone was worried but perhaps they had some similar feelings to me; this was just another setback. Everyone but my sister Cami. Her education and experience as a Nurse Practitioner gave her a deeper understanding of my condition. Don't misunderstand me though, I knew the risks, but denial and defiance are powerful tools and perhaps they even worked to keep me going and not dissolving into despair regardless of the enormity of my situation.

Soon the emergency doctor came to see us. I will never forget that moment. It is scorched into my memory forever and even now represents the moment I knew this was more than a setback, even if I couldn't accept it. He came beside my bed and with a soft sigh sat down on a stool. He looked down at his clipboard then slowly raised his eyes to mine. I read the truth in them.

He slowly explained that my brain was bleeding, again. He had been in consultation with a neurologist, and they determined it was a bigger bleed, perhaps more than my original one. WHAT!!! It couldn't be. I was worse but still okay, wasn't I? I could still think, I could still move, I could walk, albeit with more assistance. Both Ken and I were incredulous. This couldn't be!

The doctor went on to explain that he had sent the information to my neurosurgeon. The one we had met after my last, smaller bleed, two years ago. The one who had told me my abnormal blood vessel was basically inoperable. The doctor then offered me a choice. I could be admitted and stay in the hospital but there was no treatment they could offer. Or, if

Ken and I felt I could manage, I could return home and wait for the neurosurgeon to call, with the caution to return immediately if my symptoms worsened.

WAITING AT HOME

This was a precursor for so many future choices. It really wasn't a choice. I was going home, no question. I didn't want to stay another moment in the hospital. "Ken, get me out of here!" Using my walking poles and lots of help from Ken, we made it back to the car. I was morose.

More than morose, my whole being was lugubrious. I didn't want to even think I had had another bleed let alone talk to anyone else, but… my family deserved to be called and hear my voice. I put on my best mask; we all wear masks for different situations, whether it is for work meetings, a party or being polite when you are a guest somewhere. This mask is one I was all too familiar with. Telling others, it was going to be okay, it was just another setback despite my thoughts churning more than the inside of a tornado.

The sword of the inoperable abnormal blood vessel was getting too close, the thread holding it, too thin. I swayed between complete disbelief to extreme exhaustion. I was so tired. Tired of working so hard to regain skills only to have them ripped away from me again. Tired of feeling awful. Tired of telling myself and everyone else, it was going to be okay. Just tired of being tired.

Here was another choice I had to make. I could stay and languish within what life had yet again thrown my way or I could face it head on and walk the talk, the talk I had told so many others. I recalled the times I had the honour of sharing my story with others while trying to spread my message of hope – "Never Give Up! Keep Going!"

I took that day and the next to wrap myself in self-compassion and yes, feel sorry for myself a little. Then it was time to shake off my misery and start appreciating how much I had to be grateful for. I was still alive, I could still think, and with assistance, I could still get around. After the first few days, I could still make my morning cup of tea. Anyone who knows me knows how much I love my cuppa in the morning.

Ken felt this latest bleed was caused by me helping too much with the ceiling in the basement and overall, just doing too much. We could deliberate a thousand reasons why it bled again but we'll never really know. Just like the first time, we sought answers of why but sometimes there is no why, it's just because. An analogy I used before came back to me; why does a tornado destroy one house yet leave the one beside unscathed? Life is messy and full of events with no rhyme or reason. Why me? Why not me?

One person had a reason for my latest stroke. Luckily, I didn't hear about it until much later. Our band had been trying to keep together as much as possible during all the restrictions and mandates COVID-19 brought. When the weather was nice, we practiced outside but new mandates had limited even that. We all sorely missed jamming and having gigs. We had started making video calls just to keep in touch. None of us wanted the band to dissolve.

COVID-19 created many challenges and after the vaccine became available it also created many divisions, within the country, within families and within our band. Our lead singer was very much an "antivaxxer". She held this philosophy before COVID-19, but we all agreed to disagree and never gave it much time for discussion as it didn't affect our day-to-day lives. Unfortunately, COVID-19 brought this debate to the foreground.

At that time, for the world to open again, the idea of vaccine passports was gaining traction. Places were welcoming guests who could prove vaccination. QR codes were established to verify your vaccine status. We felt, as a band, if we wanted any hope of playing gigs again, we would all need to be vaccinated. Everyone but our singer supported vaccines. This caused a few heated debates on our video calls. We were at an impasse.

Before we needed to make any decisions, I had my bleed. Thoughts of vaccine passports and gigs took a backseat. Much later I heard that our lead singer believed the vaccine was responsible for my latest hemorrhagic stroke. I was incensed. What had caused my first two? Not COVID-19 or vaccines. As I said before, life is messy. On her own, our singer realized for her to stay in the band, she would have to rescind her decision and get vaccinated; her beliefs were such that she would not.

Luckily, both Ken and I were double vaccinated so we didn't need to worry about that as we knew there would be more tests and doctor appointments. We felt strongly that the best way for society to move forward was to rely on science and trust the vaccine. You only have to look through history and old graveyards to see what had happened to people during plagues before vaccines.

FIRST CALL WITH NEUROSURGEON

It was several days before the neurosurgeon called. I was feeling worse day by day. My walking was very limited. Ken took over taking Arthur out. The days were warm and sunny so when Ken was working, he would help me outside and I would sit on the edge of the patio and throw the ball for Arthur. Arthur was happy to have someone to play with although he was confused but my sudden change in conduct.

The day we were scheduled to have a phone appointment with the neurosurgeon I woke up feeling a little better, or so I thought. I slept well and felt it was going to be a positive appointment. I thought I could manage a shower by myself and even started making plans in my head for regaining my yet again lost skills.

The shower sapped a lot of my energy, and I was feeling even dizzier once I got out. I bent down to dry my legs. Suddenly, there was a roaring in my ears and my vision changed. I felt like I was churning inside a great wave, tumbling and rolling. Thud! I was on the floor. How did that happen? I was so confused. I wasn't sure which way was up or even where I was. I took a few moments to just breathe. Slowly my vision returned and the roaring subsided.

Taking my time, I sat up. I was shaking. I had never had anything like that happen to me before. I had lost complete control of all my senses and abilities. Staying sitting, I pulled on my clothes. I should have called for Ken, but I was still confused. After I was dressed, I felt like I was becoming more myself. I had my phone with me, so I called Ken. He was in the basement, that's where his office is. He had heard the bang but thought I had dropped something. I am prone to dropping items, due to my hand not working as well, so it is not unusual.

He came upstairs immediately, ready to chastise me for not calling him right away. He saw my face, saw how scared I was and just held me instead. He helped clean the small abrasion I had on my forehead where I had scraped the edge of the door during my fall. Then he got me settled into my spot on the couch and made me a cup of tea. I was no longer so confident that this was just another setback.

Not long after the neurosurgeon called. Ken was with me, ready to take notes. I told him how I was feeling and about my fall that morning. He paused (another doctor pause) and then told us the unthinkable. He told me it was time to have surgery. NO WAY! I had spent the last four years being told my abnormal blood vessel was in an inoperable location. How could he even suggest it!

Although my thoughts were like a maelstrom in my head, I let him explain his diagnosis for surgery. My latest bleed was bigger than my initial one four years ago. Luckily, it had mostly bled into the already damaged parts and my fourth ventricle. The fourth ventricle is a diamond shaped cavity in the brain stem, posterior to the pons, right in the area of my bleed. The ventricle is filled with cerebrospinal fluid and helps protect the brain.

The ventricle protected my brain and me from this latest bleed. The neurosurgeon told us if the blood had gone elsewhere the stroke would have been catastrophic. That was our first piece of good luck and good news. He went on to tell us the bleed had caused the abnormality to be pushed out a bit from the brain stem. It reduced the risk, and he felt confident he could remove it, surgically. Our second piece of good luck and news. He said I should have the surgery as I was very lucky this time but an abnormal blood vessel that rebleeds will bleed again, and next time I may not be so lucky.

Luck was again on our side as we did not need to make the decision today. First, I would need another MRI and then he could make the final determination if surgery was really an option. He would organize the MRI and I would be getting a call from the hospital soon with an appointment. We were then completely dumbfounded when he told us the surgery would be in about two weeks if the MRI confirmed it was the best course of action. He relayed all this information to us, and I felt like we were discussing someone else, not me. I had to detach myself to a certain degree to get through.

When a bleed happens under our skin, like any type of bruise, it is initially very hard, he explained. My bleed was similar to a bruise. He couldn't do the surgery when it was hard like this. But in about two weeks there would be a sweet spot of time when the blood started softening, but before it started reabsorbing. That would be the optimal time to do the surgery.

The few details he provided about the surgery were overwhelming. They would perform a craniotomy, which is a surgery that removes a piece of your skull bone to access the brain inside. He spared giving us more specifics saying we would talk after the MRI. MRI stands for Magnetic Resonance Imaging and is a noninvasive medical imaging test that produces detailed images of organs, bones, muscles and blood vessels. MRI scanners create images of the body using a large magnet and radio waves. I had many before and was still having them regularly to monitor that abnormal blood vessel.

MRI

Usually, it takes months to get an appointment as they are so busy. When Ken updated some people, they thought it would be the usual four to six months wait. It was one day. That in itself underlined the seriousness of my condition. We decided not to tell anyone about the possibility of surgery. We told them the neurosurgeon wanted the MRI completed and then he would talk with us again to determine the best course of action.

We needed time to get used to the idea ourselves. To us, it still seemed too remote despite the neurosurgeon talking so openly about it. We didn't want to worry anyone unnecessarily; we didn't think it would actually happen. Personally, I felt I had caused enough stress for those I loved and didn't want to add to it, especially if it wasn't going to occur.

We did tell my sister Cami, though. I needed someone who understood neurology and who loved me. She had a great depth of knowledge and experience. Even with her expertise, I think she was surprised about the talk of surgery. She provided us the calm we needed, telling us not to worry about it until after the MRI and my next appointment. She also advised me of some medications I could take to help manage having the MRI and my dizziness.

The day of the MRI I was feeling worse. My balance was deteriorating along with my energy. Ken drove us to the University of Alberta, Kaye Clinic, which housed many specialists, including my neurosurgeon. It also had a great imaging department. We were fortunate to be only about an hour's drive to this amazing hospital. Unfortunately, it was huge. My abilities had degraded to the point where I knew I couldn't manage walking the distance from the parking lot to the imaging department. Ken parked and then hunted down an available wheelchair for me.

I never thought I would need to use a wheelchair. Even with my last stroke, when I could barely walk, I mostly managed with canes, hiking poles, walkers, and Ken. My obstinate persistence was such I would only allow myself to use mobility aids as little as possible. Life is a journey all about learning, and I learned a valuable lesson that day, one that would be repeated many times to come. Sometimes you need help, you can't do everything yourself, and it's okay. Often, our pathway to improvement is filled with helping hands that move us along our path. I have learned and accepted the fact I needed that wheelchair, and I was grateful.

We arrived at imaging. The receptionist was very kind. She cautiously asked us if we were vaccinated, adding if we didn't want to answer we didn't have to. We told her we were double vaccinated and firm believers in the benefits and protection from them. She visibly relaxed and told us some of her harrowing experiences with people who were not vaccinated and felt everyone who was, was wrong in their choice.

Even feeling awful and filled with trepidation over what was to come with my own situation, I was surprised by the strong feelings and the divisions the vaccine was causing. I thought of our singer and her strong beliefs and realized there were more that felt the same, she wasn't an isolated case. These feelings would go on to cause even greater rifts and sadly were often joined by racist and extremist groups, further fracturing the disharmony between the vaccinated and unvaccinated.

Being distracted by these thoughts I was surprised when they called my name. It was early but I wasn't complaining. Ken, my protector and advocate, came as far as he could, telling them I couldn't walk, even though they could see I was in a wheelchair. They assured him they would take good care of me.

And they did, kind and compassionate, they helped prepare me for the MRI. Although I've had many, they don't get any easier. I had taken Gravol, to help with the dizziness. The staff placed a small pillow under the cage strapping my head down, so I wasn't quite flat on my back. As always, to manage, I closed my eyes and started saying decades of the Rosary. People may now call it meditation, but I feel blessed to have prayer for my introspection and concentration. It helps ground me, fill me with hope and gratitude and find the strength to keep going.

Again, the technicians treated me with supreme compassion after my MRI. One kind healthcare professional helped me out to the waiting room, pushing my wheelchair. Trying not to say too much, trying to respect both my privacy and the sanctity of the confidential results of the MRI, she still wondered out loud why I wasn't in the hospital. I told her I was offered a choice. Unfortunately, it wasn't my first "rodeo", and I was much more comfortable waiting for direction from the neurosurgeon at home. Ken came to meet us, and she wished me the best of luck.

The travel and the MRI completely wore me out. Ken drove me back home and I settled down for more downtime. I was feeling worse with each day. My vision was more challenging and when we watched television, I had to close one eye to manage my double vision and dizziness. I was so tired and needed help getting around. A new, very strange symptom started to develop. My hearing was being affected. So much information for our entire being goes through the brain stem and hearing was one of them. My ears randomly plugged and unplugged, and I started hearing a whole chorus of munchkins along with a single voice or sound. It was profoundly bizarre and almost held notes of possessed creatures from a horror movie. It was just one more thing to manage and try to adapt to while we waited to see what direction my healing would follow.

It was now past the middle of June, and the weather was beautiful. I appreciated getting outside. Before this previous bleed, Arthur and I had been out walking every day. I missed it. We sat outside while Ken played with Arthur, expending some of his puppy energy. Kevin and Emily were regularly calling, to check in on me and on the latest call, Kevin told us he was planning on coming and seeing us.

Being in Vancouver, we didn't see each other as often as we would like. Kevin was excellent in keeping in touch, calling almost everyday. He would arrive in a few days, having a break at school between the end of the year and before starting to teach the summer camps his school offered. It would be so wonderful to see him. With COVID-19 our visits, just like the rest of the world, had been limited to phone calls and FaceTime. I was so thankful for something other than our upcoming appointment with the neurosurgeon to look forward to.

SECOND NEUROSURGEON CALL

We were expecting the neurosurgeon to call right away. After a few days he hadn't called, and I took this as a sign that there wasn't anything he could do. It was another setback I would have to work on recovering from again. Secretly I felt relieved. It was too monumental of a decision, and I didn't have the capacity to think about it.

Ken had been trying to stay close to home, to help me, but his job had him on the road, requiring in person updates with offenders on his caseload. He had to go and have some meetings, or he would get too far behind in his work. The day he left, only for a few hours, he made sure I had everything I needed, and he would call often to check on me. Shortly after he left the neurosurgeon's office called me. Funny how that happens, it's like the old adage, "A watched pot never boils". As soon as we stopped watching, we got the call.

The receptionist called to set up an appointment in about thirty minutes. Ken wouldn't be home yet, and I really wanted him with me. The receptionist was so understanding and with COVID-19 we were all used to doing things differently. She taught me how to merge the call with Ken once the neurosurgeon called me. She was patient, went through it step by step and reviewed it to ensure I understood. I felt confident.

Next, I called Ken. He was frustrated that the call was coming through just when he needed to be away. He said he would rush and there was a possibility he would be home on time. I started to worry about him - don't rush, being safe on the road was more important than the call. I prepared myself by getting a pen and a notebook to write down anything, if need be. Again, my logical self denied any possibility of surgery while my intuition told me otherwise.

As I said, we were all used to doing things differently and virtually. The neurosurgeon patiently waited while I successfully merged the call with Ken. I was so glad Ken was there for me and I'm so grateful that my small, previous bleed brought me together with this incredibly brilliant and kind neurosurgeon.

There was no easy way to say it, so he just said it. He strongly recommended I have the surgery. He said the lesion had grown larger and was filled with blood. It was worse than my original bleed but was mostly bleeding into my fourth ventricle, keeping it from being catastrophic. Since it had bled several times now, it was riskier to leave it. He said I would probably recover from this latest bleed, but the risk was becoming unmanageable. The sword hanging over my head was too tenuous to leave.

This newest bleed also offered a gift. Since it caused the abnormality to be pushed out, it made the surgery a little less risky. The neurosurgeon felt confident he could reach it surgically. He went on to describe the surgery. I knew I needed to hear it, but another axiom, "ignorance is bliss" came to mind.

He would start an incision on the back of my neck and continue up the back of my head. He would then remove a piece of the back of my skull. Using the latest technology and microscopic assistance, he would try to remove all of the abnormality, which he depicted as capsules filled with blood. After the surgery, I would be in the Intensive Care Unit, and then on the regular neurosurgery unit for awhile.

It was a big surgery. He would have another neurosurgeon with him, and it would probably be about five hours. The brain stem is the superhighway of information for your whole being and they needed to cut into mine. The neurosurgeon told us that most people are a little worse after and I would probably need rehabilitation. He said it was like he was giving me a concussion along with another stroke doing the surgery.

There were risks but he said risk of death was quite low, only 1%. I was immensely relieved to hear that. Risks of more deficits were significantly higher, but they would probably be temporary, and he would help arrange for proper rehabilitation supports.

There was a chance the abnormality could grow back but luckily this type of abnormality was known to be slow moving and he would try to get all of it. Regardless, leaving it was riskier than having the surgery. Here we were, talking about this colossal surgery, each of us in a different physical location. It almost had a dreamlike quality to it. I felt cold all over and was starting to shake. I asked if Ken and I could talk about it and call him back. He agreed but said not to wait as he wanted to do the surgery soon, (within a week!) and it was a lot to organize.

We profusely thanked him; told him we would call in the morning and ended the call. Ken called right back and said he was almost home, and we would talk more. It seemed like only a moment had passed and Ken came in and wrapped me in his arms. We were both tearful and I was still shaky. The surgery was presented as a choice but was it really?

We just sat together and then I texted Cami, asking if we could call her. She texted back immediately, saying anytime. Both my sisters are amazing, and Cami has become the resident medical guru to all the family due to her experience and education. She is very calm, confident, and respectful. She, of course, knew I needed the surgery, but she let us talk, explain what the doctor said and come to our own conclusion.

VISUALIZATION AND DECISION TIME

That being said, she offered more explanations into what the doctor had told us and then offered us the sagest advice I would receive throughout this whole rollercoaster ride of life and death decisions. Steadily, offering us some strength, she told us about a technique she had used, visualization.

Visualization is a method of looking ahead into your future and visualizing your desired outcome. It helps to create your dream and then pursue it with faith. It is a technique that has been used successfully by athletes, entrepreneurs, and now me, someone wanting to survive and recover from my strokes and impending brain surgery.

My sister imparted her wise words; "Don't focus on the operation or being in ICU. Focus on what your life will be like in 3 months. Think about life with the malformation gone. Think about living with a reduced risk of another stroke. Focus on the good things and the good things will come." What a powerful tool. I started thinking about life after the surgery. I started thinking about how I wanted it to look and what I wanted to do.

These thoughts combined with Ken's and with all the misgivings. We still didn't share it with anyone else and we decided we would sleep on it and decide first thing tomorrow morning. My inner voice, my intuition continued to whisper in my head although the other thoughts drowned its susurrus comprehension, telling me "You already know the answer." After an evening of watching television without really seeing what was on, we went to bed.

All the questions swirled together in my brain forming an electrically charged maelstrom of unrequited apprehensions. Would I walk, talk, think – would I still be me? Neither of us slept well. When I did sleep,

I wasn't plagued with bad dreams as I had anticipated but rather broken bits of impressions not quite remembered combined with wakefulness, checking the time and listening to Ken breathing. We both woke early. I managed to make it downstairs and make some tea.

Every action I completed was laced with nostalgia as I recognized the beauty in such routine, appreciating my ability to do so. I had a growing presentiment inside my head, my soul. I felt like the decision was already made. I just had to find the courage to say it out loud, to stand behind it and make it mine.

It was a beautiful summer morning. A blue sky dotted with some puffy white clouds, birds chirping and whizzing around. The fragrance was of new growth, and dew wet grass with a hint of evergreen from our ponderosa pine. Ken and I sat together in a heavy silence, neither one of us wanting to break the peace of the new morning. With a sigh Ken said one word, "well?". That started it. He tried to tell me it was my decision since it was my head they'd be operating on. I didn't let him get away with that. This was something that affected us both. I wasn't doing this alone and that's not what Ken intended, he just didn't want to sway me initially.

Well! We reviewed some of the facts:

- The bleed from the cavernous malformation was bigger than my first stroke. The neurosurgeon informed us the way it bled saved it from being catastrophic this time. Who knew what might happen if it bled again?
- With a malformation that had bled more than once, the risks of not doing anything were higher than the risks surgery presented.
- The risk of death was only 1% during surgery. Having more deficits was higher but hopefully temporary.
- This latest bleed presented an opportunity, even a gift in that it pushed the malformation out, making a successful surgery more likely. It was a limited time offer though.
- If we didn't go through with it, we would continue to live with a sword over our heads, always wondering when it may cut me down, waiting for the BIG one.

- If we didn't go through with it, we would always be wondering what might have been.
- From Cami's advice, we visualized what would our life look like in 3 months; me on the road of recovery, being able to keep every gain I made, not wondering if and when it may be taken away again.

That confirmed it. Without realizing we had made our decision. It was a choice that really wasn't. The stars were aligning in my favour to finally be rid of the cavernous malformation. The benefits outweighed the risks. We would be foolish not to go through with it. We both had tears in our eyes but no doubts. A huge weight lifted from me along with an internal affirmation that this was right. My conscious, intellectual brain was finally listening to my intuition, and they wholeheartedly agreed.

Ken then offered his own prudent advice. This was it. This was what we were sticking to. There'd be no more discussion, no more what if's or but's and maybes or regrets, no matter what happened. We would be strong and together get through it and come out the other side better for it. I thought of a line from Disney's "Beauty and the Beast" – "Screw your courage to the sticking place". Ours was firmly fastened in our decision.

There was no feeling of wondering if this was right. I felt it right down into my soul that this is what was meant to happen. We finished our morning drinks, me my tea, Ken his coffee. Ken went to call the doctor's office. With our decision made we now recognized how much work it would be on the neurosurgeon's part to organize everything.

"There are moments which mark your life. Moments when you realize nothing will ever be the same and time is divided into two parts - before this, and after this." John Hobbes Fallen.

CHAPTER 6

DECISIONS AND SURGERY

O ur son, Kevin, was coming in a few hours. He lived in Vancouver with his wife, Alix. They had gone through university together in Lethbridge, earning both their music and education degrees. They had moved to Vancouver for Kevin to earn his Master of Music and stayed. They both loved the city and had found good teaching jobs. Vancouver also offered many musical opportunities for Kevin to grow as a musician. Alix always helped support him in his dreams however she could and herself was flourishing, entering in her own masters' program.

Kevin taught in a different school than Alix and had started summer break before her. With my latest hemorrhagic stroke, Kevin wanted to be with us, see me and help out as he could. Due to the world pandemic of COVID-19 it had been a long time since we had seen each other. Fortunately, we had all received our vaccinations already. I was so excited for him to come although the impending surgery overshadowed everything.

Ken left to pick up Kevin at the airport. The neurosurgeon would be calling again with more information about the surgery and if Ken was still out, I would merge the call again. It was a cool and useful new skill. We were both still numb but had the pervasive sense that we had made the right decision – no looking back! We'd call the rest of our families after the doctor's office called back, together.

Soon Ken came back with Kevin. Arthur, now one year old, had only been a small puppy the last time Kevin met him. Arthur provided some much-needed comic relief when Kevin came in the backdoor. Again, because of COVID-19, it had been a long time since someone other than Ken, Emily or I came into the house. Kevin entered first. Arthur happily ran to greet who he thought would be Ken. Boy, was he surprised, and more than a little scared. Arthur immediately peed a little and in trying to run away so fast he looked just like Scooby Doo trying to escape a ghost; legs running but not going anywhere. His feet finally found purchase and he came and hid behind me. I could not stop laughing. It felt so good, and it was soooo funny!

Kevin came and enveloped me in the most beautiful, intense hug. We both cried a little, not wanting to let go, making up for almost a years' worth of missed hugs. He sat down beside me in the kitchen. Without having to say anything, Kevin understood and said, "Yah, dad told me. I'm so glad I'm here."

Ken joined us and we sat around the kitchen table, catching up, overjoyed to be talking in person, not over the phone, Zoom or FaceTime. I told Kevin the doctor would be calling to confirm everything, and I had two questions to ask. I needed affirmation again that the likelihood of death was only 1% and if there was a chance the protruding malformation would shrink back before the surgery.

Arthur soon realized Kevin was pretty cool and was now his newest favourite human, wanting constant petting. It wasn't too long before the neurosurgeon called. He had gotten the message of our decision. The first thing he said was, "I'm glad you're going ahead with the surgery, you made the right decision" Any qualms we may have had were dashed away, asserting the sense of rightness. He reaffirmed the chance of death and also said the protrusion would still be protruding for the surgery, not to worry. He said he had a lot of organizing to do but it looked like Tuesday, June 29, would be the day, only five days away, his office would call.

There it was. No looking back. The figurative ball was rolling; now to let our families know. Still sitting at the kitchen table, we put the phone on speaker and started calling. Since Cami had been involved all along, we let her know the doctor had called and it was "go". I had already texted her that morning to let her know of our decision, saying I would call after we spoke with the doctor. She had been so amazing before, not trying to sway our decision but agreed with the neurosurgeon, it wasn't really a choice, this was the best course of action for my future. She reiterated the visualization, focusing on our future. Best advice ever!

LETTING PEOPLE KNOW

It's funny how you have a preconceived idea of someone. I know my sister's husband loves us, but the miles between our homes keep us from being truly close. Often, our families keep up to date on events via Cami and my conversations. Cami shared with me the concern he expressed over the decision about brain surgery. He urged her to call and tell me to have it, that it wasn't really a choice. He wanted the best for me, and he trusted Cami's expertise as much as I did. Cami resisted and let me come to my own conclusion. She told me she had a plan B in place if I had said no to the surgery.

My sister Lydia, with her heart of gold, tried to make us feel better by easing the mood, helping bring some normalcy to this untenable situation. We would chat again over the weekend. Emily was just heading into work, taking the gondola up the mountain in Jasper to work in the gift shop. We decided to call her after work. I know I would find it difficult to go to work after hearing news such as what we'd be sharing. I couldn't believe how hard it was telling people I loved and cared for, especially my children.

I know how much worry and stress I had already caused them with my previous bleeds. Logically I know what has and is happening to me is not my fault. This is just one of those things we have no control over. I've spoken about it in talks I've been privileged to share. It's like taking the blame for a tornado or a flood. The only thing we have control over is our response, how we act. I know this. But I have trouble believing it in my heart. It boils down to me; if I didn't have this malformation in my brain causing strokes and needing surgery, I wouldn't be inflicting stress and heartache on those I love. It's warped but it's hard to change what you feel.

My misguided feelings made it so difficult telling my parents. They were in their eighties and carried a lot of stress from my previous strokes. I could tell they were being strong for me over the phone, again the time between our visits prolonged due to the pandemic. It was so tough to have this type of conversation with my parents. At one point my mom had to give the phone over to my dad.

I reaffirmed the most likely positive outcome, and having previously checked with Cami, offered they could call her for further explanations. She was experienced in this field, and it alleviated some of my stress as it was difficult to hold my tears in check. Ken took the responsibility of letting our friends know. He knew I could only handle so much, still dealing with the effects of my most recent bleed as well as now preparing for brain surgery.

The last was Emily, My Wonderful Baby Girl, a nickname coined years ago when she entered her contact information into my new iPhone. We were impressed with her stoicism. Fortunately, her schedule allowed her to come for a visit before the surgery. I would have two of my children close to me, both in my heart and in my home.

But only two of my children. I'd still had no contact with my eldest daughter. The reasons were still too complex for me to fully understand. I apologized for whatever I had done to cause this, but she still needed a break. I wanted to just grab her and hold her close, knowing it might be the last time, but it was not to be.

After much deliberation, I emailed her, letting her know what was going to happen. Despite the estrangement, I will never stop loving her. A mother knows her child, even before birth there's a connection that cannot be severed even when the umbilical cord is cut. She is my daughter forever and it was my responsibility to tell her, even if there was no response. Surprisingly she did respond. In her brief reply, she wished me well and even signed it with "love". I was elated at the response. Maybe the surgery was the catalyst to bring my daughter back into our family.

PRE-SURGERY

To prepare for surgery I would need a pre-surgery physical exam by my family doctor. She had been with us since the first stroke and her support was beyond compare. She had shared her cell phone number with Ken. Ken, with his ability to get things done when needed, texted her and she stayed late after work to complete my physical.

We were the only ones in the clinic, the time being so late. My doctor, at the end of her long workday, did not rush us. She let us express our fears and efficiently helped us through all the pre-surgery paperwork from the neurosurgeon's office. After my physical was completed, she helped us organize the rest of the paperwork, including the lab work I had to get completed the next day. She labelled it urgent.

We had no idea how much needed to be done for this surgery to happen, just on our end. I can't imagine what was happening on the neurosurgeon's side. It was considered major surgery. In addition to the physical exam, I needed blood work, an ECG and a chest x-ray. With the requisition forms in hand to get the work done tomorrow morning, my doctor walked us out herself while we profusely thanked her. Again, the words seemed so small for all she had done for us.

The next day was another beautiful summer day. It seemed the weather was offering us the best days of summer early so I could take in as much as possible before the surgery. Ken had some work commitments in the morning but with Kevin home it took away some of the stress. He would take me to the hospital to get all the medical tests done.

The Wetaskiwin hospital is often very busy. We hoped we didn't need to wait too long, especially since we were still following COVID-19 protocols. My doctor had put urgent on the forms, but she said just to tell them I was having brain surgery and that would move things along.

Kevin was my advocate for sharing information. The surprise in each persons' face when told I was preparing for brain surgery said it all and reminded me of the seriousness. I was still having trouble marrying the idea of brain surgery to my brain!

All the staff were so kind and compassionate and in just 45 minutes I had all the necessary tests completed. It was amazing and perhaps offered a prognostic glimpse into my care during and after surgery. Back home we navigated the rest of the necessary paperwork and consent forms, for the surgery itself and for blood products, to send back to the neurosurgeon's office. Since my family doctor had organized and explained it to us, it wasn't too bad. Kevin scanned them on his phone and Ken was able to send it along once he got home.

Then the emails and phone calls started, more information, more forms, more questions. None of us realized how much pre-work was necessary. It was incredible and gave me a new appreciation for the amount of work being done on both the clinic and hospital's side. The questions asked were so specific, asking about my lifestyle, how much I exercised and even about my sex life. That one caught me by surprise. Later in the day we received final confirmation that the surgery would be on Tuesday, June 29, 2021. A date that will forever be burned into my memory.

Finally, the last set of forms and phone calls were completed, no more until Monday. There would be a barrage of phone calls then, varying from the admissions clerk to the anesthetist, all to help me have a successful surgery. It was incredible and a little overwhelming. They said all the phone calls could take between two to four hours. I was so glad of the support of my family. We helped each other.

Emily, having officially graduated from university, was having a very unique convocation. There was no dinner, no walk across the stage, no photos with professors and friends. All due to COVID-19. We watched, us in Wetaskiwin and Emily in Jasper, her online convocation. It consisted of regular speeches, a keynote speaker, and honorary recipients. Emily's time to shine was her name scrolling across the screen, celebrating the culmination of four years of hard work.

Bad things happen to good people. We have no control. COVID-19 was proof of that for the entire world. All we can control is our response and we respond the best way we know how. We were celebrating Emily's convocation, in our current locked- down, physically distancing existence, as best as we could. And we were responding with hope and courage to my latest stroke. I truly believe we were given a gift within all this craziness, a chance to make things better. For me, it was no choice. I would recover to the best of my ability and be okay! Period!

This was an unthinkable situation, but we recognized how much worse it could be. The latest stroke could have left me with far worse impairments or taken my life. It could still be inoperable, leaving us waiting for the next one. The amazing support network we had, both in our personal life and with the upcoming surgery, was incomparable. It was a blow, but God had softened it as much as possible while offering hope of reducing my future risks.

We spent the weekend cocooned in the safety of our home. I felt fragile and just wanted to keep those I loved close to me. I didn't have the capacity for much else. I appreciated every moment that weekend: sitting outside, sipping my tea, watching Kevin play with Arthur, and talking. I spoke with my family and some of my close friends. It was positive and the support and love flowed freely through the phone connections. We all looked to a future after the surgery, a future without the malformation. It helped me immensely.

I had considered writing a letter to each of my children but that seemed too macabre. I wasn't going to die and if I wrote something ahead of time it might influence my fate. Maybe I don't really believe that, but you never know, you put it out into the universe, and anything can happen. I wanted to attract only positive energy, so I kept my thoughts pointed in a positive direction and a full recovery.

That weekend a very special package arrived for me. It was from Cami. It contained some feel-good items, just for me, as well as a calvary of positive messages. The best was a bracelet. It was a simple, solid silver bracelet, that fit perfectly on my wrist. The best part was the inscription on the inside. In bold letters it heralded the phrase, "Keep Fucking

Going"! Life is tough, we must be tougher! I put it on and didn't take it off again until the surgery. I packed it and kept it in my hospital bag, to remind me.

Later on, Kevin and I played some music together and I shared some projects of my attempts at song writing. With his musical prowess he soon had chords assigned and played them on his guitar. It felt so good, so normal. Kevin cooked some meals for us and in no time had picked up on doing all sorts of small jobs that needed to be done. Between my latest stroke and Ken's still recovering shoulder, it was a struggle to get everything done.

THE DAY BEFORE

It was Monday morning, June 28, the day before my surgery. Ken and I started the day by taking Arthur to the rodeo grounds to burn off some of his almost endless energy. It's so quiet and peaceful there, surrounded by fields and some small marshes. We often saw deer and there were always lots of birds. The morning sun was quickly dissipating the cool of the night, promising to be another hot, summer day. I sat in the car, windows open, watching Ken throw the ball for Arthur and appreciating being outside.

Soon we were back home, ready for all the pre-surgery phone calls. If you look for the silver lining, you can find it; I was so much happier having all these appointments over the phone while sitting in my backyard with my family. Something that might not have happened pre-COVID-19. The longest call was with the anesthetist. He had a list of very specific questions, again wanting details about my physical fitness level. I hadn't been able to do much since my latest stroke but before that, barely two weeks ago, Arthur and I were out walking every day.

By lunch we were done. All done, this was it, it was really happening. Tomorrow my skull would be cut open and people would see my brain. Trying to grasp the enormity of it was, well, mind boggling. I used all the tools I could; visualization of the future without a malformation, not allowing any "what ifs" to surface and focusing on only a positive outcome all made it bearable. All this mayhem was good, it was the opportunity in the challenge.

Emily had arrived the evening before, having taken some time off from her work in Jasper. She sat outside with us while I received all the phone calls. The day was already getting hot. Ken, Emily and Kevin were spoiling me, granting my every wish. I was pretty easy to please as I just wanted to spend time together. When Kevin and Emily decided to play in the sprinkler to try and entice our water wary Arthur to get a little wet, it made my day.

I wanted to join in the water fight, running carefree while chasing the kids with the icy hose water but I was content to just watch. Arthur wanted no part of splashing water or sprinklers and soon found a good hiding spot, out of the way. Emily brought Leo, our bearded dragon out and he enjoyed the hot sun and his little homemade swimming pool, just the right size for him. He had no problem getting wet, splashing around in the water. It was a lovely afternoon.

We sat outside, most of the day, with the sun shining and the birds singing, nature injecting each moment with hope and light.

All too soon it was time for bed. Ken and I would be getting up at 3:45 AM to be at the University of Alberta Hospital for 5:30 AM. So early but I didn't think either of us would be sleeping much anyway. After many hugs and "I love you's" with the kids, we went to bed. Ken and I did manage some sleep, drifting off while holding hands.

SURGERY DAY

Soft notes from my iPhone woke me. In an instant the reason for this early rising flooded in. I was wide awake. My bag was already packed, clothes picked out, nothing else to do but wash up and head out. In no time at all we were ready. Kevin and Emily woke up to say another goodbye and good luck. Their sleepy eyes filled my heart to overflowing as I kissed their cheeks one more time. Soon, I'd be talking to them again. Soon!

Hurry up and wait. That's often the theme when something significant is pending. We were shown to our pre-surgery room. "Room" is a little generous, nook is maybe more appropriate. After an initial flurry of activity, with changing into a surgical gown, more COVID-19 protocol questions, more blood work and such, we were left alone and just waited. This was the worst. What do you talk about? Everything that needed to be said had been. We'd said more "love you's" than a whole series of romance novels. We both tried small talk but soon resorted to listening to other conversations and hearing about other people's surgery. It brought back reminders of the lack of privacy in a hospital from my stay with my first stroke.

Presently a friendly, confident young woman came into our alcove. She was holding bundles of gel pads and wires. She introduced herself saying she was a neurophysiologist. A what? She patiently explained her role during my surgery. A neurophysiologist is a neurologist with a focus on the nervous system. They attach multiple electrodes, some gels pads and some needles, to a patient during some types of brain surgeries to monitor and interpret electrical signals to ensure that critical brain and nervous system functions are not damaged during the surgery. They are an integral part of the surgical team, avoiding or reducing any complications.

This sounded like science fiction. We couldn't believe the number of specialists working hard to help me. Using a fine piece of sandpaper, she roughened my wrists and ankles and attached the gel pads. Since my surgery was in the brainstem, where so much information for our entire body is transmitted, they needed every advantage they could garner. She would run a mild electrical current through the gel pads and needles to monitor my responses during the entire surgery. The needles would be inserted once I was asleep, about one hundred of them, she said. If she noted any unusual responses, she would instruct the surgical team to immediately stop working and reassess. She would be watching out for me, keeping me safe.

On a funny note, while reading the paperwork for the surgery at home, the title "Sub-occipital craniotomy with monitoring" was everywhere. I thought it meant that they would be monitoring my vital signs during the surgery and wondered why it needed to be so clearly defined in the description of the surgery. Knowledge is power. Maybe it was better that I didn't know this ahead of time.

Her work completed she exited our alcove. We waited anxiously, hearing other patients being taken. I flip flopped between relief that it wasn't yet my turn to wanting to go right now. I just wanted it to be done. I didn't want to have to say goodbye to Ken. After minutes stretching longer than an endless horizon over the ocean, a kind nurse came for me. She was quick and efficient while exuding confidence and compassion. She had experience with loved ones and didn't allow Ken or me to become emotional by going slowly or delaying the inevitable. Ken didn't say goodbye but rather firmly told me, "I'll see you soon."

After a short jaunt, rolling along in my bed, we arrived in the operating room. I was overwhelmed with the amount of equipment, bright lights, and people. There seemed to be about ten people in there, all gowned, gloved, and masked. Everyone had a job to do, and it almost seemed choreographed. The anesthetist introduced himself, exuding confidence, and experience, the same one I had spoken with. Was that only yesterday? After questioning a dark bruise on my arm (where had I gotten that?) he put two IVs in my hand. I would have four more in my arm once I was asleep, including one in an artery.

The nurse explained I would be on my stomach for the surgery for better access to the back of my head. They would move me and shave my head once I was asleep. Again, I was amazed how quick and efficient they were. I had no time to think or dwell, which was good. While the nurse was speaking, I was starting to feel lightheaded. I told them I was feeling dizzy and that's the last thing I remember.

I AM ALIVE

Dizzy, blurry, beeping. Where was I? What were all those sounds. My eyes wouldn't open. Try, try harder. A sliver of light. Someone was grabbing my legs and squishing them, they let go, but they did it again, every few minutes. Quit touching my legs! I was so cold, a deep into-my-bones cold. Murmuring, faraway voices. A voice I recognized. KEN! He was here, I was here.

Wearily I tried to focus the swirling inside my head. I tried to make sense of what I thought was chaos all around me. Slowly my thoughts started to take form and I was able to organize them to make a coherent sentence in my head. I had brain surgery. I was ALIVE! I survived! I was ALIVE! I hadn't yet opened my eyes or even tried to speak or move but somehow, somehow, I had this resolute feeling, I was still me!

I was alive, I survived and slowly I was starting to understand I had made it through brain surgery. I heard Ken's voice. I felt him tenderly hold my hand. I was able to open my eyes and see a little light and make out some shapes. I think I managed to croak out "I'm okay." (Ken told me I also asked him to tell the kids I was okay, and I loved them.) He was there for me, always.

Then I was sick, sick to my stomach. "Was my head going to open up?" was all I could think about while the nurse got a basin in front of me, just in time. There was no sense of time, barely any sense of space. Consciousness came in and out of focus along with my vision. I was sick many times that night, made all the worse by having an empty stomach. They had used a certain type of anesthesia so as not to affect the neuro-physiological monitoring and I didn't react well to it.

Soon Ken was by my side again, had he left? Was it the next day already. I had no sense of time. I was starting to feel a little better, no longer as sick to my stomach. I was able to see a little better despite everything being double. Try as I might I could not bring my vision together. At times, it was closer, and I could ascertain what I was looking at. My legs were still being massaged and I figured out I had special stockings on that inflated and deflated as a prevention for the risk of blood clots,

Deep Vein Thrombosis. I found out later they are called Intermittent Pneumatic Compression Devices, which are inflatable sleeves worn over the lower legs after major surgery.

I was able to form more words to Ken, assure him I was okay. Even with all the tubes, stockings, catheter and other medical devices I felt I could still think. I felt my personality was still intact. I thanked God for being alive first and for still being me second. I had no idea if I had any physical deficits, but I was so thankful for the chance to find out and work on it. My resolve was such that I felt the hardest part was over, the rest would follow, all was good. My head was all bandaged up but surprisingly there wasn't a lot of pain. It was more just a feeling of numbness than anything. I was feeling better, and my stomach had settled down. I overheard conversations from the other Neuro ICU patients' nurses and thanked God anew for how well I was doing, while saying a silent prayer for the other patients' recoveries.

By the next evening I had improved such that they felt I could be moved to the Neurosurgery Ward. I remember clearly, a nurse and a physiotherapist coming in and trying to make me stand, hefting me up and supporting me in an upright position. Ken says that never happened, I was still pretty groggy so who knows. The neurosurgeon came and did some assessments while I was still in the ICU. He asked me to lift my right hand. That was the first sign that something had changed.

My hand had a substantial tremor in it. I had trouble lifting it up. But it was more than just a tremor. It is so hard to describe. Usually, when you lift your arm, it rises in one smooth, direct motion, and returns much the same way, following the instructions from your brain. I had lost control of these basic skills. My arm would move seemingly, of its own accord, taking a wild and convoluted route. The return trip would be a dramatic fall, following the path of least resistance.

I had lost control of my own muscles in my right arm. I couldn't even acknowledge the exacerbated sensory and general weakness effects of my left side as they were so superseded by the new problems on my right side. I had never had problems with my right side, it had always been my strong side.

The same was happening with my right leg. I couldn't walk. I had lost control of that leg, in strength, control, and function. I would ask my leg to do one thing and it would do something else. When I tried to command it to do a motion that it had done for over fifty years, it was like there was this vast, empty expanse where the knowledge should have been. It would perform these bizarre movements, always crashing back down with utterly no control whatsoever.

I could not walk!

THE EFFECTS FROM SURGERY

Maybe I should have been more upset. Maybe I should have lost control of my emotions along with my muscles. I think I was just too tired. And the feeling of "the worst is over" continued to grow, helping me to accept my physical deficits. I knew I had the fortitude to get back what yet another injury to my brain had taken. This wasn't over. I still had lots of fight left in me.

The deficits were surprising, but the neurosurgeon explained that it was not unusual, and he thought I would regain most of my function back quickly. He felt the surgery was a success despite my new handicaps. He explained he had removed the malformation plus another capsule of blood. I'm not sure what that meant but it seemed like a good thing to have removed it. The neurosurgeon was cautiously optimistic that he had taken away the risk of another bleed but an MRI in three months' time would be the final determination. I was still too tired and muddled in my mind to really comprehend any of it. Good thing Ken was there, my advocate and second set of ears.

Truth be told, I really hadn't comprehended the seriousness of any of this. My estimate was that I would be in the hospital less than a week and then back home. My packing reflected that belief. One of my good friends had a sister who had brain surgery a few months prior and that was her hospital experience. I was in a perpetual dichotomous situation. On one hand I knew this was the most significant of my life-threatening experiences with stroke, yet on the other hand I thought, "I just need a few days and I'll return to my old new normal." How naïve I still was! I could not imagine what recovery was going to look like but holding onto those denial-based thoughts was my lifeline for not giving up as well as my tenacity for pushing forward.

That evening they took out my catheter and I was on my way to my new temporary home. It was in the early evening; everyone was busy. Again, I found it all a little overwhelming. But soon I was in my new room, Ken helping me get settled. As he said good-bye, I felt lost despite the support from the nursing staff. I was having trouble peeing on my own and I hated the fact that I needed so much help just to pee. The nursing staff were professional and supportive, trying their best to put me at ease. It helped but the bathroom needs still bothered me in a way I needed to get over in a hurry. The next few days I had many bladder scans as I figured out how to effectively pee again. The bladder scanner was an amazing device that could tell how many milliliters of urine was in your bladder.

There are so many things I had not considered before I had surgery, peeing just being one of them. The questions, the round-the-clock vital signs checks, the total dependence on the staff for my every need. The hospital food. I still had no real appetite and barely ate anything. The plain, mushy oatmeal held the most appeal to me. Soon I was able to raise my bed more so I could drink some water, look around, and eat my oatmeal. I was always at somewhat of an incline to help manage my vertigo. I was regaining my skill of "going" to the bathroom, but I couldn't "get" to the bathroom by myself.

I still couldn't walk. At all. I was so dizzy, everything moving around me, exacerbated by my vision challenges. My right hand continued to shake when I tried to control it and I noticed something else peculiar. When I was resting, or falling asleep, my arms relaxed by my sides, my right arm would suddenly jump. Just jump right up, maybe fall off the side of the bed, hit my side, who knew. They called it ataxia or "spastic" reflexes. My right leg often made the same bizarre movements.

Ataxia is a condition usually related to damage to the part of the brain that controls muscle coordination, the cerebellum. It causes loss of muscle control and coordination of voluntary movements. The cerebellum is right in the area of the brainstem and the pons, the same area they were doing the surgery. I held onto what the neurosurgeon had said and knew with time and hard work I would overcome this and gain control over my muscles, walk again. There was no other option, I would get better, and I had the gift of being alive and having the time to do it.

The next morning, I was feeling a touch better. I still couldn't do too much, mostly reliant on the nurses for everything. My double vision and focusing my eyes continued to be a challenge. They gave me a patch for one eye to help me be able to see. It was a relief to not have to try and focus just to make sense of what was around me. I had a CT scan that morning. I couldn't move myself at all and that's when I became aware of the special blanket I was laying on.

When it came time to transfer me onto the CT table, the staff were able to inflate the special blanket I was on. It made the transfer quick and easy and reduced any jarring and bumping. I felt like I was on a cloud. They deflated it for the scan and then, quick as a wink, reinflated it to move me back onto my stretcher. All the advances in patient care are amazing and it probably helped reduce the stress on the nurses' backs too.

I managed to eat a little oatmeal after the CT scan. Food held no appeal but at least I wasn't nauseated anymore. I was using my left hand more, even learning to feed myself with it. I was compensating for not being able to use my right hand and I was making it work okay. Ken came again and sat with me. My memories for that day are still a little hazy but I held onto my stubbornness that I would improve, exceed their expectations and be walking.

The yucky, sick, completely horrible feelings would improve bit by bit. I just needed another day to rest. Tomorrow would be better. I held onto the concept of visualization Cami had shared with me. It was a powerful tool to manage those first few days when every minute hurt.

Over the next few days, I learned more about what had happened during my surgery. For me it seemed like a blink of an eye. For Ken and the rest of my family, it was many excruciating minutes, stretching into hours of waiting.

The doctors had predicted the surgery would take about five hours. With the time I went in, Ken was expecting a call by 12:30 - 1:00 PM at the latest. When he hadn't heard anything by 2:30, he started calling. After several calls all he heard was the surgery was complete. It took over six hours. Then the neurosurgeon took me for an emergency CT scan. That was it, no details. I can't imagine their anxiety, even fear, of not knowing. Something I've said before, and feel is true; it is easier to bear hardship yourself than see someone you love to have to endure.

Next Ken heard was I was in recovery and even trying to talk. I have no memory of this, I wonder what I was trying to say. Finally, that evening, I was in ICU and Ken was by my side. The faraway voices were Ken sitting beside me and the ICU nurse stationed right at the end of my bed. I was alright. Ken told me later that I wouldn't wake up from the anesthetic. They had tried different ways and when I still wouldn't wake up, the neurosurgeon took me himself for the emergency CT scan. I can attest to the many ways they tried to wake me when I discovered my entire chest was bruised.

They had attempted to rouse me using a sternal rub. A sternal rub is a painful stimulus to determine the integrity of the brain and its function. The sternum, or breastbone, is rubbed vigorously with the knuckles of a closed fist to create pain. With the amount of bruising I had, they must have been very vigorous. I was fortunate to have bruising as the only after effect of that potentially life-threatening emergency.

We kept finding more bruising. I had all six of my IVs in my left arm. It was bruised from my elbow right down into my hand. It was an alarming array of blues and purples. Ken then noticed bruising on my right jaw, just in front of my ear. Even the front of my neck was bruised, even my tongue! The nurses said it was probably a combination of being intubated and neural monitoring.

The neurophysiologist put needles in my tongue. Who knew? I have always been one to bruise easily, a real peach! The worst was all the blood in my hair. I found out later they had some type of brace on my head, to stabilize it during surgery. That made sense. No one wanted a rogue movement occurring during brain surgery. The words used by the neurosurgeon was they affixed the brace right into the sides of my skull. I was beginning to think I didn't ask enough questions beforehand, or maybe it was better that I hadn't.

Ignorance is bliss or sometimes we learn the information when we are ready to handle it. I found out later I had had two minor seizures during the surgery, adding to the explanation of all my bruises, especially my tongue. I would learn even more about events during the surgery in the months to come.

RECOVERY

Each morning a team of neurologists and neurosurgeons came and saw me. Sometimes it included my neurosurgeon, always some residents, who knew who else? They introduced themselves but I didn't always catch the names flying by. I just knew there were many ambitious, well-educated people, all there to help me. I had usual checks of my orientation to time, date, place and my name then some tests of strength and coordination. Several days after the surgery they came prepared to remove my bandages. I was in no hurry to have them removed. I felt the dressing was probably keeping the incision safe, especially since I was spending most of my day lying in bed.

But it was time to come off. I remember the doctors telling me the bandage was stapled right to my scalp. They weren't the same as staples used on paper, these staples didn't curl in, just straight down. I was curious how it would be removed and a little nervous. I slowly sat up in bed and the doctor pulled out what looked like a pair of wire cutters. I leaned forward and in quick, efficient moves, he did something to the staples and without warning, zip, pulled the entire bandage off. I was surprised how quickly it came and how little I felt. The whole back of my head was numb, lucky for me! The doctors all leaned in and told me it looked really good.

That's the unfortunate part, I couldn't see any of it. Again, maybe it was lucky. I asked about sleeping and lying in bed. They told me it was fine to lay back on my head. It made me nervous, so I tried to turn my head while laying, taking direct pressure off the incision. I reached back and carefully felt the back of my head, avoiding the incision. My head was so numb. The pain I felt was to the right of the incision, at the base of my skull, towards my ear. It was very swollen and tender.

Shortly afterwards, Ken came in. I told him that my bandages had been removed. He wanted to see it but also didn't. He didn't know what to expect. Neither did I. After a few minutes he had a look. He didn't look long. It was not a pretty sight. The incision was about eight inches long, starting in my neck and continuing up the back of my skull, slightly towards the right. It was sutured with a unique seam called a running stitch. I had used a similar stitch in sewing. My good friend Lucy had told me it was called a blanket stitch. They had only shaved what they needed off my head. From the front you couldn't even tell.

Ken took a picture for me. I was very curious. I was taken aback by the sight. My first thoughts, and words, were, "Frankenstein!" That's what it reminded me of. Ken sent pictures to Cami, no one else. This wasn't something you could share with just anyone and Cami had the experience not to be shocked by it. He had previously sent pictures of my bandaged head, telling her the bandages were stapled right into my scalp. She was a great resource for Ken, to further explain things, offer comments on the incision, allay his concerns. She and Ken had a laugh, expressing they never ever would have considered they'd be sending texts about staples and stitches in my head!

I kept my focus on the future; I would feel better, this was temporary. I still wasn't eating much and knew I needed to. I ate my oatmeal and forced myself to try the fruit cup on my tray. Since my first stroke most fruit held a salty, bitter taste. But this was soft, something I could probably manage, and I needed to eat. Ken opened it up for me and I tried the apple blueberry sauce. It was cold and easy to swallow. There was not much of any taste, but most importantly no salt. There was a hint of fruitiness, just enough to become my next favourite food after oatmeal. Oatmeal and fruit cups! Look at me go.

Another anomaly that I noticed was my vision had changed even when my eyes were closed. Typically, with closed eyes, I see patterns, or dull lights behind my eyelids. It would move about slowly. I think this is something most of us see when our eyes are closed. After my first stroke, a busy day would cause it to swirl in a circular pattern on the backdrop of my lids. For the first few days after surgery, I noticed a strange vision. When my eyes were closed, I now saw a solid backdrop of a greyish coloured wall, almost like concrete. It was unyielding, sturdy, flat. This wall maintained itself, unchanging whenever I closed my eyes. It seemed so real and solid I felt that I could reach out and touch it, feel its smooth, inflexible surface. It lasted for several days until eventually the old patterns and lights returned, slowly breaking through the rock fortification. Maybe it was the first of many walls I needed to navigate during my recovery. Or maybe it was built from all the medication delivered into my veins during the surgery.

The next day Ken arranged for Kevin to come for an outdoor visit. First, a nurse helped me wash up. I was looking forward to feeling clean and hopefully getting some of the blood out of the hair they hadn't shaved off. I knew I badly needed a wash when the neurosurgeon asked me if I had just showered, my hair so greasy it looked wet. I needed considerable help to wash up and my nurse was full of gentle compassion. I felt much better and this time my hair really was wet!

Getting ready to visit with Kevin, one of the unit staff found me a wheelchair we could borrow. Ken was the only one allowed to visit me inside thanks to COVID-19. Emily was heading back to work, but we usually had more opportunities to see her. She would be braving the long drive from Jasper and be coming back soon. Kevin was heading back to Vancouver. He did plan to come again in August but who knew? I was excited to see him and some different scenery. It would be my first trip out of my room.

One of the many hard-working, kind nurses found me a pair of pajamas instead of just a gown. It felt good to wear something more reminiscent of clothes, even the cotton hospital pajamas, stamped with the Alberta Health Services logo. She helped me change and wrapped a warm flannel blanket around me. The weather was summer hot, but my body still held a chill from the surgery. Ken brought me out of the ward after the nurses assisted me into the wheelchair. Ken, his previously dislocated shoulder still bothering him, was able to manage the wheelchair. I found the trip a little overwhelming, still weak and wobbly, but determined to have a visit with Kevin.

I was enveloped in a hug filled with so much love it brought tears to my eyes. Kevin held me tight, the relief coursing through his arms and right into my heart. We were both here, able to appreciate the gift of each day! We found a quiet spot in the shade. Ken asked Kevin if he saw the back of my head. Kevin said he was avoiding it. He did eventually look, agreed with the Frankenstein reference but recognized it was only temporary. He termed it "Franken-head". Kevin noticed the lack of control on my right side as well but otherwise he was amazed at how well I was doing. The weather was warm, and the visit was incredible. I was so thankful. I had survived the surgery. I was here and I seemed to still be mostly me.

All too soon it was time to say goodbye. The brief outing and visit tired me out, much more than I expected. Ken brought me back to my room and helped me back into bed. It was time to rest. Rest, such as it is in a busy hospital is an ephemeral thing. I was lucky to have the far bed, by the window. I could turn and look outside a bit and felt I had a little more privacy. Still, you can hear almost everything about everyone else. There is a bond between roommates. We learn so much about each other, being privy to conversations with doctors and family, just because there is no other choice. There is a level of respect for this knowledge and an unspoken agreement to keep confidentiality.

"There are many truths of which the full meaning cannot be realized until personal experience has brought it home." J.S. Mill

CHAPTER 7

HOSPITAL LIFE

After my rest I felt a little better. I was managing a little more food and was given a menu where I could choose some of my items. Oatmeal and fruit cups were still my mainstays. Later in the day I was able to text my family. Ken had been keeping in contact with them, sending them pictures and updates. It was a lot of work for him and now I was up to doing a little of it myself. It felt so good to text with them and soon I would be calling. I was so blessed and grateful for all the love and support. I would get better! I owed it to them. I owed it to myself.

A very special text came in later that day. Kevin and Emily know my love of music and especially my love of listening to their music. Emily, with the voice of an angel, studied Vocal Performance and Opera in university, while Kevin is a musical genius in his own right. The two of them worked together and made a recording of Celine Dion's "My Heart Will Go On." Kevin laid several tracks of different instruments he played while Emily added her incredible singing. There I was, sitting in my bed, with the typical organized chaos all around, crying my eyes out with shear happiness, as I listened to their love and caring pour out through the recording. My roommate heard it and added her tears to mine. Some things are so exceptional they are beyond words.

The next few days developed a kind of rhythm, vitals check, doctor check-ins, questions, meals, medications, blood work. Unfortunately, blood work often came between 3:00 and 4:00 AM. Sleep is not a priority for the patients. No wonder patients need to nap during the day. They don't get any sleep at night. How did it come to be that bloodwork at 4:00 AM was a good idea? I'm sure it woke my roommate up as well. Every night at the U of A, 4:00 AM bloodwork.

To ensure the right patient got the right care we all had our own QR code on our hospital bracelets. We would be scanned before any blood work, or any medications were given. They would scan the vials for blood collection or the packages for medication then scan our bracelet, if it matched, all was good. The information would automatically be on their computer. A nurse rarely came in without their computer, like a dog on a leash. Cami had told me when she was working, they called them COWS, Computer On Wheels. A fitting acronym.

The most challenging aspect was waiting to be helped to and in the washroom. Think about a time you had to go but had to wait; it can be quite uncomfortable, sometimes almost excruciating. I remember reading a part in a book about an officer interrogating an elderly woman. His second in command was ready with torture implements but the officer had another idea. He kept serving her tea. When her bathroom needs became unbearable, he got all the information he required. An interesting tactic. I don't think it would work on Rambo!

My stressed bladder needed relief and sometimes I just couldn't wait. Ken was often with me. After having to wait too long several times, I said to him, "Just grab the commode and help me. I can't take it anymore." Like the amazing husband he is, he did. Not the first time, and certainly not the last, I was testing the 'In sickness" part of our wedding vows.

Since I was a fall risk and couldn't walk, the nurses had enabled the alarm on my bed so if I tried to stand up, or fell out, an alarm would sound. I wasn't going to try but a few times the nurses forgot to disarm it when helping me to the washroom; it was loud. The first time, Ken didn't turn off the alarm and got in trouble from the nurse. "But I had to go pee!" He ended up helping me more than once but always remembered to turn off the alarm after the first time.

We saw how busy the nursing staff was. They weren't stressing our bladders on purpose or using interrogation tactics by making us wait to use the bathroom. We heard the bells from all the other rooms, calling for a nurse to help them. Bing, Bing, Bing. I'm sure the staff heard bells in their head when they went home after a shift. Often, some of the nurses would be working on several units. They would fly in and out of our room. You became adept at calling out for anything you needed if a nurse even came close to your doorway.

Being a patient is a loss of independence and privacy. You are at the mercy of someone else for all your needs. I knew the staff cared for me and were caring but sometimes, busyness just got in the way. Caring for sick or injured people is a challenging job at the best of times but during a world pandemic? I can't even imagine how tired the staff were. But sometimes they forget what it's like to be a patient. One prime example was an experience with my night nurse, of course after Ken had left for the day. I was on very little medication, even for pain I was only having Tylenol. I dislike taking medication, and avoid it if I can, although I know sometimes it is very necessary. That night, the nurse came in and told me to get ready for my needle of a blood thinner. She spoke as if this was a common thing.

Blood thinner?! A needle? I had never in my life taken one. I have always had thin blood, with a low red blood cell count and low iron for much of my life. To intensify this, my neurologist and neurosurgeon had both advised not to take anything with a blood thinning effect because of my abnormal blood vessel and hemorrhagic strokes. Even the anesthetist advised against anything with blood thinning qualities when we spoke on the phone before my surgery.

Now this nurse was casually telling me to get ready for a needle, in my stomach, that would thin my blood. I assumed it was a mistake and told her so. She double checked and said no, I was prescribed this, and she needed to administer it right now. There was no explanation of why or how it came to be I required this needle of a blood thinning medication. For four years I had been careful to avoid anything with a blood thinning effect. I refused the medication. I would not let her inject me with it. I was recovering from surgery and a brain injury; the conversation made me feel like crying. I was adamant though. NO!

The next day, another nurse and a doctor came to see me. They explained I had been prescribed the medication because I couldn't walk and was recovering from major surgery. It was protocol to administer this medication to reduce the risk of blood clots. They took the time to explain it in detail and answer any of my questions. It made sense and they made me feel at ease. There would be no risk of another brain bleed, especially since the neurosurgeon had removed the malformation. I was still getting used to the idea of life without the malformation.

With this explanation and the reassurance of no risk of another brain bleed, I submitted to the injection. I still wasn't thrilled about it, but the explanation made sense. This interaction reminded me of the important work I was a part of on the Patient, Resident and Family Council with Covenant Health. Through our work we were advising on improved patient engagement while elevating patients to be a valued partner of their own healthcare team. I wanted to be a part of the team, not just a submissive automaton programmed to obey.

STILL BEING A PATIENT

It's often the little things that mean so much to you when you are a patient. It's amazing how much you can hear when the room door is left open and how much light comes in. The small act of closing our door after a nighttime check, drawing the curtain between our beds, giving us some privacy in the bathroom, asking what we need instead of assuming, speaking to us, not around or above us, shutting off lights that you have turned on is priceless when you're a patient. These little things make such a huge difference in maintaining our dignity. Some things are not little, like ensuring the commode is lined up over the toilet. After being made to wait, sometimes hours, before being able to relieve yourself, you realize it's going all over the floor. It is beyond embarrassing.

Rationally, I understand there is more need than capacity, but it doesn't make it easier. While lying in my bed, ruminating over the needle ordeal, and seeing the flurry of activity around the unit I had a vision of what this hospital life compared to. I needed to release the impression onto paper. Here is my surgery brain-addled reflection of life in the hospital. It took me awhile to decipher what I had written. I think I had mostly used my left hand. It is interesting where my thoughts went during this time of total dependence.

Life as a Patient:

The ebb and flow of the routine. As predictable as the ocean tides, yet as serpentine as all the rivulets of water either escaping or encroaching. You're in the safe little cocoon of your bed, a non-descript curtain for your wall. Shift change, vitals check, mealtime. The same questions, ensuring you're okay.

- "Can you tell me your name?"
- "Do you know what day it is?"
- "Do you know where you are?"
- "Do you have any pain?"
- "Squeeze my fingers, bend your knees, push your toes."

Always the same, as the busy seabirds fly in and out, already looking towards the next wave.

"Stop, wait, can I get some water? Can you help me to the washroom? I dropped my pillow and can't reach it."

Too late. Independence shredded; dependance multiplied. You limit how much you drink, time it for when you think you'll be helped to the bathroom. The teacher has been a bursting bladder too many times. Your loved ones have arranged your things, all is within reaching distance so you can access it without asking. You dig deep, rely on memories of happier times and your steadfast belief that happier times will come again. You push yourself to make a slow, uncoordinated exercise routine to convince half of your body to start working again. This is only temporary, a necessary setback towards the higher goal. You can endure, you can make it, you can ride this tide. Soon, you'll be moving with the ebbs and flows, riding the waves, catching the surf, instead of succumbing to the powerful currents of a dependent routine.

My little tirade of hospital life is no reflection on the nurses and aides that helped me and every other patient. Let me be clear about a few things. They were doing their best despite being at the inconclusive end of a world pandemic that had stretched on for more than 17 months. They were trying, often being short-staffed, being ordered to work in more than one area, being ordered to work a double shift because of not enough staff. Often, they were late to help me because they were dealing with a potentially life-threatening emergency.

Despite all the crazy chaos I still felt cared for, I knew they were trying. They were always kind and showed compassion in their limited time. It's understandable that sometimes, in all the organized mayhem, they forgot what it's like to be a patient. Several times I commented that the government and powers that be, collecting their nice salaries and pensions, needed to come work for a week on one of these units. Running this way and that, answering bells, questions, multitasking, working multiple units.

As a healthy able-bodied visitor, Ken sometimes helped other patients. He would bring my roommate some water, grab something just out of reach. He even bought her word search and crossword books when he brought me some, to help with the long days of isolation. When we were out of the unit, patients sometimes needed help to access the vending machine or other things just out of reach. Vending machines aren't designed for someone in a wheelchair. There were lots of little things and Ken was always ready to lend a helping hand.

The government should lead by example and use servant leadership as a model. The people actually doing the work are the most important and the "leaders" are there to support and assist to ensure the workers are able to do the best job possible. Unfortunately, it seems politicians of integrity are about as common as common sense and as you look from one to another, they all kind of look the same.

I had some physiotherapy at the hospital. In their stretched too thin time, they only had time to see me twice. Another example of more need than capacity. One of the therapists shared with me a harrowing story of life as a healthcare professional during a world pandemic. She had been redeployed as COVID-19 security outside of a COVID-19 Intensive Care Unit.

She told me stories of abuse from patients, families and "anti-vaxxers". The most chilling was her recount of watching COVID-19 patients go into ICU only later to come out in body bags. I made sure to thank her for her hard work. Another conversation I overheard highlighted the abuse healthcare staff had to tolerate. A mother, not much older than I, was assisted by an aide to talk to her adult daughter using her iPad. The daughter was loudly complaining about healthcare staff and the exaggeration of the seriousness of COVID-19 saying the restrictions were just part of some government conspiracy. The mother tried to stop her daughter's rant but just didn't have the energy. The staff graciously ignored the offensive vitriol and kindly helped the mother.

With their lack of time and resources I was fortunate enough to have three therapists help me get out of my wheelchair once. With a transfer belt, a railing and lots of support I was able to stand up. It felt so good. To my surprise, we tried walking. They were right there for me, encouraging me, holding me up, and assisting me, literally every step. I managed almost 3 meters. My right leg was very erratic, even more so than when Kevin had noticed it at our visit. One therapist placed a weight around my ankle. With that and by sliding my foot along the floor, I could make it behave. All too soon it was over. I was so grateful to have had this opportunity and it gave me even more confidence that I would be regaining my lost skills. They gave me some exercises to practice on my own.

And practice I did. I could now manage to pull myself up and sit on the side of my bed. I was careful not to set off my bed alarm AND not to fall! While sitting up I had a view outside, all very downtownish looking, but outdoors, nonetheless. It challenged my vision, but I added it as another exercise. My double vision was improving, and I didn't have to rely on patching one eye as often to discern what I was looking at. Just hold on Christine, keep working hard, this isn't permanent, it will get better; it IS getting better.

Ken came every day. It was the bright spot in the miasma of medical mayhem of the neurosurgery ward. Ken would sit with me, we'd catch up, as best as we could with everyone else able to hear us. He would see if there was anything he could get for me from the nursing staff, ensuring I had what I needed. After those needs were met, he would rustle up a wheelchair and help me into it. Then we were off to explore.

OUT AND ABOUT AT THE HOSPITAL

The U of A hospital was huge, we were in one unit, on the fourth floor. With COVID-19 restrictions still in place, there weren't a lot of visitors, but still we liked to find quiet places. Our favourite was the Healing Gardens. A previous doctor and his family were the impetus for the beautiful repose within all the sickness and sadness congruent with a hospital. We could talk freely, through our masks, whilst taking in the flowers and greenery. While finding it we went through some darkened hallways, closed up for the evening, the workers taking a break from their long days. We liked these quiet areas, away from the constant hustle and bustle of the unit.

We would also go outside, although it was sometimes a longer walk to find tranquility, away from the crowds and smokers. Ken never complained about his shoulder while pushing me along, finding the perfect spot. He was still waiting for an appointment with an orthopedic specialist. I loved these moments outside. I was always an outdoors person. That was one of the reasons I loved my pre-first-stroke job so much. I usually spent part of the day outside.

Even in the middle of the steel mill, which covered more than ten acres, I found connections with nature. There were many bunnies hopping around. I should be more specific. Bunnies conjure up a vision of cute little Easter bunnies, sitting in harmony with baby ducks. These were wild hares, or jack rabbits. They were bigger than our previous dog, little Twinkie, who was a Shi Tzu. In the spring, we would often see the males fighting. Sometimes we could hear them growling. Not long after the fighting had ended there would be baby bunnies hopping this way and that.

We always had a few pairs of geese, building nests and proudly walking their children down the craneway, guarded by the load checkers and crane operators. Once we had a delay on an order of rebar because of a robins' nest, snuggled in between the bundles of 20 Metric rebar. The customer had to wait until the chicks fledged for their product. Finding these connections has always been a priority. At home we have lots of birds, sometimes a squirrel and occasionally a martin, (a type of weasel). The only animals that receive no welcome in our backyard are cats. Too many times we had found the aftermath of a feline visit in the form of a pile of feathers. Ken rose to the task, buying a soft air gun to scare any cat brave enough to stalk one of our birds! With the addition of Arthur, few cats dare to invade our property.

Our brief outings on the hospital grounds gave me a taste of what I was missing and would return to! I continued my own exercise regime and was noticing slight improvements. I started writing in my journal and was surprised how challenging it was; just holding the pen, even just picking up the pen. I persevered and kept trying to write, taking the words from my brain and placing them on paper was very cathartic. The adage "chicken scratch" would have been a compliment, though. It was a start and turned out to be a cryptic puzzle to ascertain what I had written.

Mastering my right hand was something I never had expected I would have to do. It was so natural to use my right hand, it was my automatic go to. Several times, the nurses handed me my medications in a small plastic med cup. Without thinking I tried to grab it with my right hand. I couldn't hold onto the cup and the pills would fly. We all caught on and I would grab it with both hands. Being dropsy became the new normal. My phone, a book, my food, trying to drink, we laughed at the clumsiness. But it was more than just clumsy. My brain had to develop new connections. Previous ones had been severed and recovery was a process of relearning and repetition.

Rehabilitation and exercise are the best ways to recover from any loss of function. In brain injuries, recovery and improvements can happen for the rest of your life but there is a sweet spot in therapy, usually within the first few months where gains seem to happen at an accelerated pace. Surprisingly, my speech, which held moments of hesitation and slurring, was vastly improved. Something in the surgery gave me back almost normal speech. The brain is so mysterious.

My neurosurgeon, suspecting I may need therapy after the surgery, had already put in a request for me to be transferred to the Glenrose Hospital. The Glenrose Hospital is a world-class rehabilitation hospital. It is the largest comprehensive tertiary rehabilitation hospital in Canada. Services offered included not only stroke and brain injury but also amputation, autism, burns, spasticity, spinal cord injury, and pediatric services. They boast cutting edge technology, innovation, development and academic teaching. They would come and do some assessments to see if I would be accepted.

I had some trepidation over going to the Glenrose Hospital. It was world-class and I knew I would get all the care and rehabilitation I needed but I had had a negative experience there after my first stroke. I went for an outpatient visit, hoping for some exercises to help with my vertigo. It didn't go well. The roller coaster of life is full of twists and turns. It would be unfair of me to judge this amazing hospital from one unfortunate incident. It would be like judging Disneyland because of one bad hotdog!

The next day two well-dressed young men came into my room. It was a rehabilitation doctor and a resident from the Glenrose Hospital, ready to complete my assessments. The resident looked just out of high school. You know you're getting older when the young adults start looking so young. They were very kind and right in my room they started assessing.

It was very gentle and manageable for me but determined the significance of my new right-side deficits and the depth of my double vision. They also discovered my eyes would start shaking and moving in odd directions while I tried to track objects. There was a funny moment during the assessment, a story I like to retell. The resident was testing the amount of spasticity in my right leg. It was just like my right arm uncooperative, lacking control and full of spastic, unexpected movements.

Strangely, when he tried to induce a reflex with his little red, rubber hammer, my leg didn't move. He squatted down in front of me and tried tapping different spots. Phbwack – suddenly my leg shot out like a bullet from a gun. Right into the crotch of the crouching resident. I was mortified. To his credit, his only reaction was a muffled grunt. His partner commented that he would be a lot more careful of his position in the future while the resident assuaged my apologies by telling me it was an occupational hazard. As bad as I felt I still found myself stifling a laugh. I couldn't wait to tell Ken about it.

There were other moments that offered bouts of laughter. As I said before, our room was like a sound funnel. It seemed we could hear every word from every nurse and patient on the unit. One morning I overheard an interesting exchange between two patients. Both patients were male. I learned to recognize the voice of one as he was very loud and gruff. Also, he didn't mince words while boisterously sharing his thoughts. On this particular morning another male patient was calling "help me" from his room. My roommate and I could tell that the nurses had checked him, and he wasn't in need of actual help but who knew what was going on in his mind. I was in the neuro-ward. He repeated this request many times. Boisterous Patient had enough of the plaintive cries and yelled back, "Shut up." It continued like this:

"Help."

"Shut up"

"Help me"

"Shut the hell up!"

"Please, help me."

"Shut the hell up, nobody's coming!"

The exchange continued for a good 5 minutes. The nurses did some magic and both patients were soon quiet. Such is life as a patient.

My initial assessment from the Glenrose was complete and I hoped my leg to crotch incident wouldn't reflect on my acceptance. The doctors told me I was a good candidate, but they would take it to the head of their program and let me know. Despite my physical deficits my ability to think, feed myself and use the toilet with help gave me some advantages and could affect my acceptance. Again, I was grateful for these attributes but hopeful I would be accepted. I felt like I had interviewed for a new job. They even called Ken, saying I would have to work hard if I was accepted. He assured them the problem with me would be the opposite, not taking enough time to rest. He knows me well.

CHANGING HOSPITALS

The next day, the head doctor from the Glenrose Hospital came. He did a few more assessments and then told me they would accept me. I felt a great rush of relief; I got the job! He told me they would take me in either the stroke or the brain injury unit. I technically had a stroke but the type of blood vessel malformation I had, and the unique brain surgery, either unit would suit my needs. I didn't care, I just wanted to walk again and was thankful for the chance for the intense rehabilitation offered by the Glenrose Hospital. He also said it could be a week or more as they had a waiting list of people needing service.

This was far longer than expected. I had already been in the hospital for over a week. More than a week! How many days since I had brain surgery? It seemed like a lifetime ago but at the same time only moments had passed.

The next day one of the nurses casually mentioned I would be going to the Glenrose Hospital in three days. What? She thought I knew. She went and double checked. Yes, they had received word about my departure just that morning. I think my neurosurgeon had something to do with speeding up the process. He was really looking out for me.

Ken was happy for me. I was thankful yet very nervous. It was another unknown. My roommate had just come from the Glenrose Hospital and shared her positive experience with me. It helped but I knew I was safe where I was. My first stroke had increased my anxiety and how I handled it and since the surgery it had increased even further. I also just wanted to go home. I was very self-motivated. I would work hard no matter what. Did I really need this? Yes, I did, I couldn't walk, I couldn't get to the bathroom by myself. I needed help to wash up and shower. The list went on. Logically I knew I needed it but, in my heart, I just wanted to be home.

Conversations with Ken really helped to calm my anxiety over the impending move. Then they told me I would be transported by ambulance and their suggested length of stay was four to six weeks. My worry skyrocketed again. To everyone else I was able to put on my brave, everything is alright mask. I downplayed my apprehension while bolstering all the benefits of rehab at the Glenrose Hospital.

Again, Ken offered the words and comfort I needed. He could see through my mask and offered the words I needed to hear. He continued to visit every day, thankfully since he was the only visitor allowed. COVID-19 meant isolation for many patients. We often went to the healing gardens. The peace and quiet was a much-needed respite from the busy, noisy unit. We could also talk privately, something the room was sorely lacking.

The day before I was to go my neurosurgeon came to check in on me. He knew I was leaving. I believe he had quite a hand in getting me there so quickly. He was confident things would improve quickly and I'd be walking again in no time. I was very happy to hear that, especially the "quickly" part. Especially after the rehabilitation doctor from the Glenrose Hospital told me my stay would be between four to six weeks. I was in denial about the time frame, believing it would be 3 weeks, maximum. Even that seemed too long.

He checked my incision and asked the usual questions on how I was feeling. I would see him in the next month or so, after I was released from the Glenrose Hospital, for a post-op visit and then have another MRI in about three to five months. That MRI would determine if they were successful in removing the entire malformation. I couldn't entertain the thought of it not being successful. In my mind it was just a formality.

As he was leaving, he wished me luck at the Glenrose Hospital and asked if I had any questions. I had only one. How did they reattach the bones in my skull after the surgery? I was very curious and had no idea. He described how they cut through the skin and muscles, pulled it apart and then cut out a window of bone from my skull. Once they were done, they put the bone back in place and fastened it with a titanium plate and screws. I had a titanium plate in my head? Again, how did I not know this beforehand?

I was assured that titanium would not beep at the airport or interfere with upcoming MRI's, it was a non-ferrous metal. I was still in a little bit of shock. Not a bad shock. Just a disbelief that I had only now found out I had a titanium plate in my head, more than a week after my surgery. It didn't really bother me and maybe I even found it a little fascinating. I was looking forward to telling my family about it.

When telling my sister Cami, she immediately referenced the song "Titanium" by David Guetta featuring Sia. I used the reference in one of my Twitter posts – "You shoot me down, but I won't fall. I am Titanium!" That's me. Stroke, you keep trying to shoot me down but I'm not going. I won't fall! And I have the mettle as well as the metal to prove it.

After my initial surprise wore off, I thought back to my days when I started at the steel mill. I first worked in the chem lab, using a mass spectrometer to test the steel as it was being made. The main ingredient of the steel was scrap metal, but specific elements were added to bring it to the right grade. If titanium was required the operator would always add it close to last, when they were almost ready to pour the batch, shaping the molten metal into billets. I would race to test it, ensuring the percentage was within the specifications. Titanium oxidizes easily so care needs to be taken. In the right amounts, it enhances the quality of the steel being made. Just like me, with the right amount of therapy and rest, I'll be the best I can be.

Christine Holubec-Jackson

"Keep looking up and things are bound to follow the same direction." CHJ

CHAPTER 8

ANOTHER HOSPITAL

Soon it was my day to go. They told me the transport was scheduled for 9:00 AM. Ken had helped me organize all my stuff the night before, ensuring my clothes were within reach. Not only my greatest supporter, but he is also my greatest promoter too. We wanted to share our children's book about stroke. He helped me to sign, in my messy, childish print, several of our Glia Girl books to give to the ICU and surgery units. "The Adventures of Glia Girl, When Stroke Strikes", was the perfect gift for these healthcare heroes who worked with stroke survivors every day. I was unaccountably shy handing out these books. Thank goodness Ken took the lead or nary a book would have been shared.

The next morning the nurses helped me to the washroom early so I could be ready. I had breakfast and managed to dress myself. It took quite a while, but I did it. This was the first time since my surgery I wore real clothes. I had only worn hospital pajamas for the entire eleven days. It felt good, normal, but just putting on my own clothes really tired me out. The nurses offered to help but, of course, with my stubbornness, I refused. I was glad for it though. It gave me a taste of the independence I would soon regain.

Hurry up and wait. That was the theme of the day. The first message told me the transport would be arriving at 10:00 AM. Next message, 11:00 AM. Then lunch came, but no more messages. Ken was upset as he planned to meet me at the Glenrose Hospital. There was no point in him coming to the U of A as who knew when the EMS would arrive. I was feeling more apprehensive by the minute and secretly hoped they wouldn't show up. I was safe where I was. I knew what to expect.

At 7:00 PM we received word that the transport would be there around 8:00 PM. Almost twelve hours late. I understood the situation. They weren't making me wait to be mean. It was the same problem as with the nursing staff, more need than service. I called Ken and we decided he would just come the next day. It would be bedtime by the time I got there. It made sense but it heightened my apprehension. I was still hoping it would be further delayed, extending my stay in safety.

They arrived about 8:30 PM. Two uniformed and very professional looking paramedics came in with the typical stretcher bed, or gurney, seen in all the emergency shows. They exuded positivity, while joking around, apologizing for being late. My fears slightly loosened their grip. Saying goodbye to everyone, I held on tight to the stretcher as we began our excursion to the awaiting ambulance. The trip was exciting yet challenging. More than ten days after my surgery I was out of the hospital, embarking on the next step of this journey of recovery. Managing the movement, laying in a bed facing the back, the lights, the noise, were all overwhelming for my symptoms. For the most part I kept my eyes closed.

The paramedic in back with me was amiably chatty and the trip went quickly. He also shared the common story of too much demand without enough capacity. They were stretched just as thin as the hospital staff. He told me about the ambulance itself and what it was like to be a paramedic. He then mentioned Edmonton had a stroke ambulance. That perked me up.

Before Ken and I took a break from producing our podcasts, we had the privilege of interviewing a neurologist who was part of a team that brought in a stroke ambulance to Alberta as part of a pilot project. It was the first one in Canada. A stroke ambulance can perform CT scans, right in the ambulance. They can also administer medications that may help mitigate the effects of a stroke, such as clot busting drugs. It includes paramedics as well as a nurse, a resident neurologist and virtual technology to conference with another neurologist. It saves lives and can potentially reduce disability; Time is Brain! When we did the podcast, it was just a pilot project.

The conversation helped the trip fly by and kept me from dwelling on my dizziness and apprehension. Soon we were at the Glenrose Hospital. We breezed right in, the hour being late enough that the COVID-19 security had left. I was soon being presented to the stroke unit. The staff did not seem pleased to be getting an admittance at 10:00 at night.

Or was it just me? As I was expecting the worst, were my own fears infusing false attitudes onto the staff? It was like the movie "Snow White". She collapsed from fear in the forest from imagined terrors but when she took a moment to really take in her environment, she found it full of kind woodland animals. If Snow White could find the courage, so could I. I took a breath.

Just as with the surgery, there is a lot of work in being admitted. Questions, forms, tests, more questions. It seemed endless and I felt like crying. No! I gave myself a firm shake, got out my shovel and started digging out of my own anxiety. I smiled, I asked them how they were and mustered as much confidence as I could. My new roommate still had family with her, they were saying some prayers together which I found calming.

We weren't quite done yet. They helped me to the washroom. With the nurse standing right there and exhaustion from the trip I was again having trouble peeing. Back to the bladder scanner. Luckily this issue soon resolved itself. Then I had to be tested for MRSA; Methicillin-resistant Staphylococcus Aureus is a bacterium that causes infection and is resistant to many antibiotics. MRSA is always a concern in hospitals. Anyone coming from another hospital needs this test because of the insidious problems the resistant virus can cause. The MRSA test was similar to the COVID test, putting a long cotton tip up both nostrils.

I thought we were done, but no. I was so tired I wasn't even sure what was going on. I'm sure they were explaining it all, but my ears weren't hearing. A nurse shone a bright penlight into my eyes. He casually mentioned my pupils were different sizes. That woke me up! Was I alright, was I having another stroke? His casual attitude and response saying it was not a big deal due to where I had my brain surgery took the edge off my fear, but I asked about my pupils at all vitals check for the next several days. All the nurses had a similar response, but I wasn't fully relieved until the day they told me they were equal and reactive.

While I was still fretting about my pupils, a nurse suddenly pushed spoons full of water into my mouth. What the heck? Before I could ask or barely even swallow, in went another one, then another, then another. Eight times. I was struggling to keep up but somewhere in my tired, injured, and addled brain I thought, "Oh, they're making sure I'm not at risk of choking while swallowing."

Stroke can affect the muscles involved in swallowing. Aspirating food is a real hazard, one risk they were making sure I did not have. I passed and then another nurse explained some type of mumbo jumbo about the information board behind me. I wasn't even aware of it. I think they were asking permission to write down my personal information and therapy schedules on it. I agreed. They put a pen in my hand and told me I needed to sign a form. I could barely hold a pen, let alone write my name. I usually do a fancy signature, full of swirls. No one could tell where my first or last names started or ended but it was unique to me. I have no idea what I wrote, but I think I managed a somewhat recognizable "C".

Having an advocate for you in the hospital is so important. I was fortunate that the nurses were professional and took the best care of me possible. I was confused, tired and had just had brain surgery eleven days ago. I would have received the same thorough treatment but the presence of someone who knew me and could answer a few of the questions would have alleviated a lot of my stress. Due to government decisions related to healthcare funding, my transport circumstance made that all but impossible. Ken never made it, the hour being so late.

Eventually we were done. I let Ken know I was settled and signed off. I know he felt bad he couldn't be there, but we were both practical and the situation was anything but practical. I was exhausted. Then I had the best sleep of my life; nope. Have you ever been so tired you can't sleep? It has happened to me several times in the past, mostly when I first started at the steel mill and was working twelve-hour shifts, rotating between day and night shift. I tried to read a book; one I had read many times before. I did not have the energy to read something new and my eyes weren't cooperating. I managed to shut my eyes a little and felt a bit better in the morning.

SETTLING IN AT THE GLENROSE HOSPITAL

The nursing staff came with smiles and good morning greetings. Breakfast was served and it was similar to the food that was offered at the U of A. Except for no accompanying tea, I enjoyed my breakfast of mushy oatmeal. The staff introduced themselves, offered to help with any breakfast containers, asked if I needed help with anything else, bringing in fresh ice water without me even asking. It was a slower and calmer pace than the U of A. The staff had the time to talk a little and ask if you needed anything instead of calling out as they fled from the room. Although busy it was not the breakneck speed laced with emergencies of my previous unit. The best part, I wasn't made to wait to use the bathroom!

Another benefit was the bed itself. It was a nice, newish hospital bed with controls for adjusting the head, the middle, the overall height. It was fantastic. The most amazing part that I and my roommate appreciated, as her bed was the same, was how quiet it was. At the U of A whenever we adjusted our bed, the older beds sounded like a garbage truck compressing a full load. It was unbelievably noisy. These beds, barely a whisper. It's incredible what you appreciate, and I really did!

I was pleased to learn I would be receiving two different therapies that day. I let Ken know and he decided to come a little later once I was done. Again, with COVID-19, things were restricted, including family members attending therapy. The first was Occupational Therapy, (OT). I met with a very friendly, efficient therapist. She said my first week would mostly be assessments to create a baseline of my abilities and needs.

The tests included activities like picking up square blocks from one container and placing them into another. It should have been easy, but

I think I managed to get 6 out of 20 moved over. A few of them went flying across the room. I was disappointed to see how deficient my right arm and hand were. At least I knew my starting point. I would be the hardest working and most dedicated patient. I would improve in leaps and bounds. But first, I needed to gain control over that right arm and hand.

The porter took me back to my room. I marveled at how efficient and on time everything was. They already had a wheelchair, just for me. It stayed in my room and even had my name on it. Ken wouldn't have to go begging or searching to find one for me. The porters were organized and on time. They helped me transfer in and out of my wheelchair. This was like a five-star hotel, well maybe not quite, but still pretty good. I had my lunch and then a porter took me for Physiotherapy, (PT).

The first test was determining if I could stand. With help, yes! It was such a good feeling to stand up. Being barely above 5'2", I've always felt short. After being in a wheelchair for so long, I felt as tall as a towering poplar when I stood up. It was an amazing sensation. I will never again complain of being short.

The physiotherapist conducted several other assessments and as with the OT, my score was fairly low. I was given a weight again, for my right foot, to help control its spastic movements. This was only a starting point. There were a few more rungs than we thought in the ladder of recovery. After my move to this new hospital and restless sleep, I was tuckered. I had time for a little nap before Ken came.

The Glenrose Hospital was a little further and it took Ken at least one hour and fifteen minutes to travel to see me. Two and half hours, round trip, if there was no traffic. I appreciated his visit so much. He got to see my new abode and brought some tea. I was still tired but optimistic about the next part of my journey. Soon I'd be home.

I got to know my roommate. As I've said before, you form a special bond with your roommate. Very quickly you learn a lot from the conversations you overhear, as much as you try not to. Although it was a much larger room, privacy was lacking, and the slightest whisper carried throughout the area.

She had come just a few days prior to me. We started some conversations, usually lying in our respective beds and through the flimsy curtain that offered the illusion of seclusion. I learned she was from Africa and English was her third language. She was amazing. She seemed similar in age to me. Despite our cultural differences, we found kinship through our shared stroke experience and our dedication to our families.

She was an amazing woman and very positive. She always had a smile and always asked the staff how they were. We were very compatible, being respectful of our shared space and trying to be as quiet as possible during the night. Soon we met each other's families, extending our hospital friendship. Her daughter always came to help and bring her traditional food. It was comforting to have her next door, someone to always say good night and good morning to.

STARTING THERAPY

Soon it was Monday, Sunday being a day off from therapy. The assessments continued. Through the assessments it was determined where my deficits were. The only way was up. No choice, I would improve, I would be walking out of here. Digging deep and not entertaining any other outcome was, and is, my saving grace. When I was tired and felt like crying, I gave myself a little nudge and tried one more time.

Let me be a little more specific. I'm not a warrior, just a survivor. I know how and when to push myself but the years since my first stroke have taught me valuable lessons. I can recognize when to push and when I truly need a break. I still have naps or at least quiet times, lying in bed. I must or I won't make it through the day. I still get emotional. Tears develop and trickle down with ease, at the slightest provocation, more so when I'm tired. I have tenacity but I feel it is a keener tenacity than before. I usually can recognize how much get up and go I can muster before it's gone.

Fatigue is a real issue with stroke or any brain injury survivor. It's as real as double vision or one-sided weakness and can be a barrier to daily living. It is unlike just being tired. I am very familiar with being tired. Our busy, pre-stroke life was jammed packed. I remember one weekend where I was at work on a Saturday after a full week at work. I worked all day then drove to a venue where our band was playing a gig. We got home from the gig at 2:30 AM and then were at church for 8:30 AM to attend mass as well as play music for the service. This type of schedule was not atypical. We could manage it and the accompanying tiredness was tolerable. Stroke fatigue is a completely different animal.

Post stroke fatigue is common, yet it is often under recognized. It is bone deep weariness that is not ameliorated by rest or sleep. Just as every stroke survivor is unique so is the fatigue they experience. For myself, I would be working in therapy and suddenly have the overwhelming need to close my eyes and lay down, no matter what I was doing. It is a more demanding desire than passing up on your favourite cookie, fresh from the oven, when you are absolutely famished. One of my roommates during my hospital stay told me she sometimes had to tell her family not to visit as she was just too tired to sit with them and talk.

It was a relief for her to be able to share her concerns. No one gets it like another stroke survivor. We see the sky as the same unique colour, no longer blue. Post-stroke fatigue is distinctive. The intensity of the tiredness does not seem to be related to the severity of the stroke either. Many survivors say fatigue is one of the most difficult and distressing aftereffects they must manage. One study reported that 50% of stroke survivors said weariness was their biggest challenge.

Why fatigue is so prevalent, and problematic is not entirely understood. When we were still doing our podcasts, we were privileged to interview a stroke neurologist who shared his expertise and experience on post stroke fatigue with us. It was a fascinating interview, and the information was so valuable. My first stroke nurse helped us arrange it and sat in on the interview. It was amazing and was made all the more so by an inspirational experience they shared.

They had recently treated someone who had suffered a stroke. Their recovery looked very promising, and the survivor shared that they suspected it may be a stroke after hearing one of my speaking engagements. I had shared my story during a women's retreat and included the life-saving acronym FAST. This survivor was able to react quickly and get the necessary help for the best possible outcome because of me sharing my story and FAST. FAST stands for Face Arm Speech Time, referring to typical stroke symptoms as well as treatment, call 911 quickly. Have I mentioned, Time is Brain? Approximately 1.9 million brain cells die every minute a stroke is left untreated, that's an unbelievable number! I've heard of another acronym since, that describes my more prevalent symptoms – BE FAST, which includes Balance and Eyes.

The stroke survivor relayed the information of what I had shared during my talk with the neurologist treating them just before we interviewed him for our podcast. It seemed almost divine. We all had tears in our eyes. It was an incredibly special moment. We are all students, and we are all teachers. My life mission, even more so now, is to help others. I had always said if I could help even just one person, I would be happy. Now I want to help more, many more. Through my desire to help I find myself learning just as much, probably more. I adhere to a quote I heard, "The best way to help yourself is to help others." I tried to find who originally said it as many people have said something similar. With the number of similar quotes related to helping others, it must be good therapy, something we should all strive towards.

At the Glenrose Hospital, my roommate and I found comfort in our shared challenges. I told her all stroke survivors shared a bond, part of an exclusive club. We hugged each other and discussed some hurdles common to many stroke survivors. We both felt better for being able to talk candidly. Throughout my stay at the hospital, I had many opportunities to talk to fellow stroke survivors. Everyone's story was as unique as their stroke and recovery, but stroke was the twine that bound us all together.

With most patients spending a longer time at the Glenrose Hospital and it being a somewhat slower paced hospital than the U of A, we got to know each other's visitors. Our premier had announced that Alberta was "Open for Summer", a premature nomenclature that failed spectacularly. We were allowed two visitors instead of just one as was the case when I was at the University Hospital. Introductions of patient's families were made, names mostly remembered, care and encouragement always freely given. Since it was a stroke unit, we knew we were all there for the same reason. We could talk freely about our challenges and what we did in therapy that day. And we all understood, to some degree, what each of us were going through. We would cross paths in the hallways, the atriums and during therapy.

KEEP GOING

Every day, I attended my different therapies. I felt myself improving a little each day. My old, Type A, busy personality still exists under the years of being a stroke survivor. Every now and then it resurfaces with alacrity. I'm still me to some degree.

Way back when, in my pre-stroke life, there's a perfect example of my tenacity, or perhaps stubbornness. I was getting ready to teach a water running class. I loved it and we had a lot of people who also loved it. I was moving some equipment across the deck to get ready. One piece was a portable pool slide. As it pushed, it suddenly snagged something and jumped back at me. The bottom ran over the top of my big toe. I, of course, was in bare feet.

I felt myself turn white, the hairs standing up on my arms. I looked down and the recalcitrant slide had ripped off my big toenail, mostly. It was hanging on with the barest amount of tissue. I left the slide where it was and went into the office and sat down. What was I going to do? Class started in fifteen minutes. I was the only one there. There was no time to get another instructor.

Against better judgment but a sure sign of my personality I decided I could still teach it. I taped the toenail back on, taped my toes together, put on my water running shoes and taught the class. It wasn't my best idea, but I made it through, and no one ever knew. Back home, Ken gave me all the sympathy I needed. Taking off the tape was almost worse than the initial injury.

My stubbornness is definitely still intact. But I truly believe that it's what has carried me through. All these traits whirl together to make me one stubborn, never-give-up, wanting-to-beat-the-odds, kick-ass survivor! "Keep Fucking Going!" (I still had the bracelet in my bag, to remind me every day!)

Every therapy session, I gave it my all.

"Do you need a rest, Christine?"

"Not yet."

"Do you want to try standing for the next exercise?"

"Yes!"

"We're done for today, great work."

"Already? Are there some exercises I can do on my own time?"

This might appear contradictory after talking about post-stroke fatigue. I push myself but now I know how far. I know when to stop and have a rest before I feel sick or start crying, which sometimes is the only way I can express that bone deep exhaustion. The therapists caught on and ensured I took appropriate breaks but didn't hesitate to correct me. I needed it. Often, I didn't even realize I was compensating for my deficits.

The first most common one was closing one eye to manage my double vision. Necessary to prevent me from running into a wall, not good when we were doing eye therapy. "Open your eye" Oops! The second was scrunching my shoulders up. This one would happen when I was trying to get my legs to work, concentrating on right hand exercises, standing practice, just about any rehab. "Relax your shoulders," I'd be admonished. Oops, again. I appreciated the reminders. I didn't even notice I was doing these things. There were many more but those two happened just about every session.

The therapists know how to get the best out of their patients. There were times they suggested an activity, like standing independently while hitting a balloon back and forth. Were they crazy? Balance was a huge concern; did they forget I was a fall risk? But they wanted to try it, so I was game. Before I knew it, I was doing it. The simple game we used to play at the kids' birthday parties became a valuable physio exercise. Of course, the therapists had considered every possible hazard and took steps to mitigate it. But that was a few weeks down the road.

First, I learned how to maneuver my wheelchair by myself. Again, the skills needed just for that were something. I used a combination of my foot and my hands to push myself along. I have a whole new respect for people who play wheelchair sports. The strength and skills needed are tremendous. The first time I went to a therapy session on my own was so exhilarating. I had to navigate the hallways, use the elevator, remember what floor I had to go to, and then take the right hall to the physio department. Even with my vision challenges, I only ran into a few things. Renewed independence was starting to blossom.

After all the exercises and hard work I put into being able to move my own wheelchair, whenever I see someone using a wheelchair or any mobility aide, instead of feeling sorry for them because they are reliant on an aid, I'm going to say congratulations because I know the work it takes to get to the point of moving yourself. Being able to use a wheelchair or any mobility aid takes effort and skill. So, WAY TO GO!

My room was on the third floor and therapy was on the second. Initially, using the elevator made me nervous. I was anxious that I'd be too slow and get caught in the doors. The hospital elevators had lots of sensors to prevent just such an incident, but my irrational fears endured. I'm happy to say, I never even got close to being squished by those sliding doors. I also appreciated how steady the elevators were, no bumping or jarring or even butterflies in the stomach feeling. I'm sure many stroke and brain injury patients have troubles with dizziness, and I was happy they took care to have smooth elevators.

Being at wheelchair level, I also started noticing something peculiar once I was in the elevator. Someone else, who was wheelchair height, took the time to stamp shoe prints on the metal, sliding, elevator doors. The size made me think it was a man wearing some kind of running shoe. One day there were two prints, usually the left foot. The next day a whole line of shoe prints.

It was always the same shoe and foot, left. I pointed it out to Ken, and we started keeping track of the prints. We also discovered that between the three elevators available, the prints were mostly in just one. The cleaners were kept busy wiping off the prints from the stainless-steel doors but just as soon as they cleaned them, the shoe print bandit readorned his signature design. Ken and I found humour in the situation, although I'm sure the cleaners did not. I was tempted but never once added my own unique tread. Maybe I've watched too many episodes of CSI and didn't want to get caught.

After maneuvering my own wheelchair, next was being able to transfer in and out, independently. We practiced sitting to stand, stand to sit multiple times, shifting to move from one seat to another, sometimes from differing heights. I was very motivated. Standing up after being wheelchair bound was exhilarating. It's a feeling like nothing I've experienced before. As I mentioned before, I'll never feel short again after spending time always at wheelchair height.

Relearning the skill of transferring in and out of my wheelchair was particularly liberating because it meant I could finally use the washroom on my own. Just imagine having to always ask for help to use the washroom. That was one of the things that bothered me the most. Not only was I asked at least twice a day if I had had a bowel movement, the staff knew every time I went since they were right there with me. There was an utter lack of privacy and a total need for dependency. I was a prisoner of my own shortfalls, but I persevered and gained a little more autonomy, securing the privilege of using the washroom independently. I felt like William Wallace in Braveheart – "FREEDOM".

SHARED BOND

This is another aspect of life in a rehab stroke unit. In any other crowd, if you mentioned you achieved the honour of using the washroom on your own you would get funny looks, at a minimum. Here, people understood the significance and immediately congratulated you. In talking to one survivor, he shared the funniest story. While determining if he could be independent in the washroom, a nurse encouraged him, saying "Good job!" He laughed when retelling us saying it had been a long time since he had been praised for wiping his ass. Such is life in rehab.

We all encouraged each other as much as possible. We shared in regained skills; we cried about real life hardships. We supported each other in accepting the unimaginable reality of stroke. In the hospital it didn't matter who we were before stroke, lawyers, teachers, housewives, rich or poor. We were all in the same boat, stroke was the greatest equalizer. Being a stroke survivor means navigating life after. It is truly life altering. It can touch every part of your life including driving, your home, mobility, career, income, and so much more. Every day we saw each other, being warriors in overcoming these obstacles, making impossible decisions, trying our hardest. It was and still is inspiring and humbling.

One survivor needed to make the hard decision to sell her home, give away her dog and apply for assisted living. Another survivor's husband was on the brink of collapse as the experts recommended his wife move into long term care. One survivor had a young child who was too scared to come into the hospital. These were the everyday challenges faced in one way or another by all of us.

Bad things happen to good people, and I realized anew that as bad as things were, they could be so much worse. Therapy was going well and each day I learned something new and not just new exercises. Often, a new exercise delineated a challenge I haven't even recognized. The therapists were remarkable, and with their expertise and toolbox of activities were able to isolate just what I needed to improve; a shaky muscle, uncooperative fingers, wandering eyes.

The therapists followed a very organized route through recovery, one activity building on the next or targeting specific deficits. I often thought, "What a silly exercise, why do I need to put clothes pins on a yard stick." Then I tried to do it. It takes a surprising amount of skill to pick up a clothes pin, open it, then reach up and pin it onto something. It challenged my right hand, it challenged my reaching, it even challenged my vision. This one seemingly simple exercise.

There were many similar exercises and I needed all of them. They gave me some supplies, such as a band to stretch between my fingers, a ball of putty to squeeze, weights for my ankles, and more. I was able to practice during my down times. I usually had about two and a half to three hours of therapy a day. It may not sound like much but when you are recovering from a stroke, you need the rest; remember the stroke fatigue.

The part of Occupational Therapy that I disliked the most, meaning I needed it the most, was vision therapy. Yes, there is such a thing as vision therapy, and it can be very intense. With my double vision and wiggly eyes, it was very necessary.

Double vision is termed "diplopia". If a stroke affects either the visual pathways in the brain or parts of the brain that process visual information, it can affect how you see. It often happens if there is damage to the cranial nerve three which is located in the brainstem. It can affect the nerves and muscles that help control eye movement and assist in keeping the eyes aligned. It can also affect how your brain interprets the information your eyes are sending to your brain. Together these were causing my double vision as well as eye movement troubles and perception.

During assessments, at both hospitals, they discovered my eyes often wouldn't move correctly. They would be jerky in their movements, not move together, or one eye would just wander off. This is called nystagmus. In OT, we did many vision exercises. One was trying to find different sticky notes stuck to the wall with letters or numbers written on them. Another was tracking a little pink ball on the end of a stick. One that I found really tricky, was termed eye stretching. The therapist would put the pink ball on the edge of my field of vision. Without moving my head, I had to stretch my eyes to look at it and hold for five seconds. My eyes didn't like that one. We started with one eye covered. Eventually it improved but it always left me feeling like I spent one too many turns on the merry-go-round.

The occupational therapy also helped me regain full function with my right hand. As I mentioned before, it would move spasmodically, and I had trouble controlling my movements. My right hand liked to curl down and out with my fingers starting to enhance my Frankenhead look. The therapists had their toolbox full of exercise and gave me a whole workbook I could use on my own time. The workbook consisted of exercises that encouraged pen or pencil use. It started off with practicing making shapes, starting with straight lines to wavy lines to circles, eventually leading into the cursive alphabet. I had to use my left hand to help my right hand hold the pen properly and then work I did, until either my hand or my eyes had had enough.

PRACTICE THROUGH DAILY LIVING

There were lots of opportunities to practice throughout the day too, just through daily living skills. Brushing my teeth was one. Most times the toothbrush would go flying or I couldn't hold it well enough to effectively brush. I often used my left hand, even though it was weaker. The therapist gave me a foam tube grip to put on the handle. The extra width and soft surface made it easier. I still had to concentrate but with practice my teeth were well brushed, and the toothbrush stayed in my hand. The hospital bathroom was designed for people who had mobility issues and it was much easier to access the sink and toilet from a wheelchair than at the U of A hospital, which was designed for people who were standing.

There were plenty of other chances to practice just through daily living. One of my favourites was playing Hangman when my youngest daughter, Emily, came to visit. As I said, due to COVID-19 change in protocols, hospitals now allowed two designated visitors. I had to approve them as visitors, and they went through a COVID-19 security check every visit. Only Ken and Emily were designated and only one at a time was allowed inside. Emily was driving back and forth from Jasper, to visit. She was getting tired of being away from home though.

Although being in Jasper, living in the mountains and working on top of a mountain was exciting, she was starting to feel like she wanted something more in line with her degree. Vocal performance in opera was her major, and her minor's included history and culture. Emily has a talent for finding jobs and was soon hired into a new position. She found one in a museum, not too far from home, being a museum educator as well as developing programs. She was moving back home.

It all seemed to happen very quickly. For me, being in the hospital, it held a feeling like reading the headline news stories. I was not very involved and unable to help at all. Despite that, I was glad of it. I am a worrier and all that driving back and forth fueled my fear. Soon she was back home and one of my designated visitors.

Back to Hangman! Emily would help me in my wheelchair to one of the quiet atriums. It was always nice to get out of my room and the hospital provided several beautiful areas for patients and staff to spend time in. Hangman is a fun word guessing game. One player draws the gallows, complete with a noose, and provides a word for the other player to guess. For every wrong letter guess, another part of the unfortunate victim is drawn. The only salvation is the word being guessed before their whole body is drawn!

It's a great game, one I played with my mom and was happy to pass onto my own children. Emily and I had always enjoyed it, even using scraps of receipts found in my purse whenever we found ourselves in a waiting room for something. Now it provided even more than a fun way to pass time. It offered a whole slew of skills to practice akin to my therapy. I had to focus my eyes, hold onto a pen, try to draw a noose and a victim, print letters, think of a word to either guess or have Emily guess.

It's almost mind-blowing when you think of all the steps and skills in simple tasks or games, we consider common place. I was relearning many of them and had a new appreciation for what I had previously taken for granted. Emily was very patient and would always retrieve the pen when I dropped it and didn't rush my slow printing, drawing, and guessing. We had lots of fun, making the most out of our time together.

"Wisdom comes from experience. Experience comes from life's trials and tribulations. Surviving those events gives us strength. It is a beautiful circle of learning and living" CHJ

CHAPTER 9

WALKERS AND WEEKENDS

Another practice I did on my own was practice my bass guitar. Ken had brought my first bass to the hospital. It was smaller than my regular bass, being called a Micro Short Scale. It was still a good size and somewhat heavy. Ken set it up for me in my closet, on its' stand. I was able to maneuver my wheelchair to get it. I was very nervous, with all my right-hand deficits. My left hand only seemed to have some general weakness and the usual sensory concerns, the comparison to my skin feeling like burning ice being the best description. I did and still do wear an extra layer on most of my left side to try and appease the unpleasant feelings.

I was able to sit in my wheelchair, holding my bass. I could play! Not well, and very slowly, but I could PLAY! It was very important to me. I love playing music and being part of a band. I concentrated and was able to move my fingers to practice some basic riffs I knew. Most of the fundamentals were still there as well as the muscle memory. I practiced most days, growing new connections in my brain. Slowly my fingers started cooperating. If my bass was still out when one of the porters came, it was always a conversation starter. Even though the bass was small, it was still cool, being bright purple. I could only manage about five to ten minutes before my brain overloaded and shut down, resulting in fingers not working at all. I couldn't hold a pick yet and with my ears still wonky, if I listened to music on my headphones, it all sounded out of tune.

As with all my deficits, I knew it would only get better. And I knew how to compensate. Also, Ken and I watched many music documentaries, and many bass players never use a pick, so it wasn't as much of a priority if I couldn't get back to using one. My bass playing restoration was up to me, my attitude and dedication to practicing. I would get it back, I had to. There was no way I was going to be replaced by another bass player in our band.

Practicing my bass always brought memories of our one podcast, "Don't Forget Me", with Canadian rock legend, Alan Frew, from the band Glass Tiger. As I said before, we were so blessed with each and every one of our guests. Alan Frew was also a stroke survivor. There was a connection between him and a friend of my eldest sister, Lydia. She arranged for the interview when his band was performing a concert in Edmonton.

I was so nervous. Alan Frew was used to performing in front of thousands of people and just speaking with him made my anxiety soar. A few questions into the interview and I forgot my nervousness. We recognized we were brethren, both part of an exclusive club only for stroke survivors. He spoke candidly about his stroke and recovery. As an added bonus, we got to watch his concert later on that day. They are an amazing band and as a novice bass player myself, I appreciated the talent. They must have hours of practice under their belts.

Just like practicing and improving with each podcast we did I improved every time I practiced my bass. There was something unique and cathartic about putting on my headphones, listening to a song and playing along. I was getting my groove back. I was seeing success in regaining other skills too. Every day in physio I practiced standing, my balance and walking. Soon I was practicing with a two-wheeled walker. Previously I hadn't understood the difference between a two and a four wheeled walker. A two-wheeled walker provides more stability and won't move as quickly. There are only wheels on the front legs. The back legs usually have a smooth surface or, maybe tennis balls with a slit cut in them for the feet to go into.

WALKERS

With only two wheels, it is easier to handle. It's perfect for someone with mobility issues or like me, relearning how to walk. They are only meant to be used indoors. The back legs with the tennis balls wouldn't slide very well on sidewalks. After lots of practice in therapy I was given one to use on my own. It stayed with me in my room and even had my name on it. I was still a fall risk, so I was also lent a transfer belt. This was so I could practice with staff or Ken aside from therapy.

Part of me hated the fact that Ken had to help me with therapy while another part loved the fact that Ken was there for me and helped without question. I think it was that I needed therapy at all. There was still that part of me, that control freak, independent, type A personality that had a lot of trouble asking and accepting help.

My tolerance was wearing thin. I just wanted to be able to do things on my own. These thoughts carried a pall that threatened to overtake my ability to keep going, to focus on a better future, that shrouded my hopes with despair. My first reaction whenever I felt these waves of anguish starting to break in on my consciousness was to retreat, isolate myself. I tried to be kind to me. I wouldn't succumb to pity but allowed recognition that I had been through a lot, was still going through a lot. I tried to practice self-compassion, and usually engaged in an activity that brought me some comfort, or at least filled my brain enough to displace these dark feelings.

I was rereading a book about a very brave woman who had overcome almost insurmountable hardships several times in her life. The most recent one carried a very significant injury causing a permanent, life-altering disability. It is a very inspiring book. She was and is consistently very brave, always using visualization about where she wanted to be. She never shied away from the hard work presented by her disability. I wish

I was more like her; I have times where I doubt my recovery and lament over what has been lost to stroke. Stories like hers help to replace any morosity with gratitude and gumption.

Ken always came to the hospital with a good attitude and something special for me. He bought me some new clothes, perfect for therapy and someone who couldn't manage buttons or zippers. He brought me tea, snacks, anything I wanted. He took home some of my clothes to wash and always brought the freshly washed ones and put them in my small bedside dresser.

He was always getting me something, including things to cheer up my area, making my stay a little easier. He and Emily had purchased two live flowering plants. They were beautiful and brightened up my windowsill. Alongside my live plants family and friends sent flowers. It was almost like they had planned their flowery gifts. When one bouquet was nearing its' end another one showed up. For my entire time in the hospital, I had beautiful flower arrangements gracing my windowsill. I was grateful for the natural freshness and happiness they brought.

Our friends and neighbours at home didn't forget about Ken either. They were helping him with yard work, bringing over home cooked meals and treats. One neighbour we didn't know as well even baked him a pie. My sister Lydia ordered Ken several weeks' worth of "Hello Fresh" meals, to reduce the workload of shopping and deciding what to cook for meals. We are very blessed with the many people in our lives who care for us.

The therapists had given me many exercises to complete on my own. I completed them diligently. Some I needed help with. One of my goals was to walk out of the hospital under my own power. I knew walking completely independently was perhaps a little too much, I was still using a pole when I had my latest stroke in June, but if I could leave with just a walking pole, that would be the icing on the cake. Ken supported me in all my goals, and he wanted me to walk almost as much as I did.

After we visited a bit and I drank the tea Ken brought, I would get into my wheelchair, and we would head out. Ken brought my walker and transfer belt. I was on the third floor, but we headed down to the second floor. Many of the therapies offered at the Glenrose Hospital were on the second floor. After supper, the therapists were done for the day leaving the second floor quiet and almost empty.

I'd park my wheelchair, Ken would put on my transfer belt, and thus began walking practice. Ken had been invited to one of my therapy sessions, learning how to help me and manage my fall risk. We'd walk around the hallways, the building being somewhat circular. There were many intersections leading to various other therapy rooms, and I never quite figured out where we would end up. Ken had a better sense of direction. Slowly I went from five meters to ten then thirty, taking rests when needed. There were lots of chairs placed strategically around the hallways. One evening, Ken was encouraging me to keep going, I was ready for a break, and I tried to insult him but instead of calling him a "Drill Sergeant" I called him a "Lion Tamer!" We both laughed and I was able to go further while Ken imitated a whip sound.

We would sometimes see the evening cleaners, greeting them while trying to stay out of their way. We would also peer out the various windows. Many of the windows possessed bat-like gargoyle creatures just outside. They seemed medieval and an accompanying shrill bird call enhanced the impression. We could hear it through the thick glass. As we pondered over these strategically placed effigies, we concluded they were for scaring away pigeons. It was more fun to imagine ourselves in a stone castle, looking for some ancient hidden treasure that would restore anyone who touched it to full health.

All too soon it was time for Ken to go home. This was the longest time in our entire marriage we slept apart. Often, we fell asleep holding hands. I knew he'd be back the next day, but his departure always left a little void that I tried to distract myself from with crossword puzzles or other such mind games.

ROUTINES

I am very routine orientated, especially when I'm by myself. To pass the time in the evenings I would juggle managing fatigue and therapy. I was tired, but I didn't just want to watch a show on my phone. I became scheduled to the minute. I would do one crossword puzzle, one word search, then I would read for 15 minutes. By then the nurses would have come in for my evening vitals check. After that, I would change into my pajamas, then I would watch a show.

During the day I downloaded shows from Netflix or Emily's Disney Plus account. I only watched movies I had seen before. I found watching anything new too hard for my eyes and brain to follow. I would watch a show for just over an hour, while enjoying an evening snack. Then, sleep. This routine helped me to feel like I had some control over an uncontrollable situation. Everything in my life was regulated by hospital life. Having control over these little sub-routines helped me immensely to appreciate the help and expertise staying in the hospital offered.

Hospital life has its own rhythm, synchronized by the huge responsibility of caring for many individuals with a whole smattering of medical and personal care needs. It is overwhelming to think about all the organization that must happen for a patient to have all their needs met. Just meals alone. Meals were more work for staff thanks to COVID-19 as all meals were eaten in our rooms instead of a common area. We were offered limited choices, but choices, nonetheless. I wasn't forced to eat pork or the proverbial bread and water. On a side note, there is no physical reason why I can't eat pork. I just never have nor ever will like it. Even as a child, I really never liked it. My mother always teases, saying I can't really be Czech if I don't like pork. (Both my parents are Czech). If I was starving, I'd eat pork!

My unit alone had approximately 30 patients. There were two more units on my floor and two other floors of patients. That's a lot of people to feed. Most of the time, my orders were correct. There were a few little hiccups. One morning, my entire breakfast, tea included, was ice cold. The nurses quickly helped, and I ended up with two cups of hot tea (I was in heaven). They were apologetic but I realized, and voiced my thoughts, that I was lucky to have someone trying to bring me food I had chosen. Mistakes happen. When I saw the food delivery people, I always greeted them and tried to thank them for their hard work.

The funny thing about the food schedule in the hospital was the timing of meals. All our meals came within an eight-hour window. Breakfast at 8:30 AM, lunch at 11:30 AM and supper at 4:30 PM. It was a pretty quick turn-around. I wasn't that hungry by lunchtime, but I soon learned it's a long time from 4:30 PM to 8:30 the next morning. I always saved a bit from my lunch and supper to have for my evening snack with my show.

I was probably one of the few people who liked hospital food. Maybe it was my lack of sense of taste, but it was good. I missed fresh food but, on the whole, I had few complaints. Breakfasts were the best and when I got home, I spent time figuring out a recipe to make one of the items, blueberry rounds, once I had recovered enough to bake again. Sunday nights we would get a sheet with the options for the week laid out and we just put a tick beside our choices. It was repetitive but I could pick what I wanted. It was easy, no figuring out what to make, no cooking, no clean up. I would listen to an audio book while I ate. I quite liked mealtimes.

WEEKENDS

Weekends were for relaxing. I found this frustrating as I wanted to get home as soon as possible and thought I should have therapy every day. I did my own therapy on the weekends with the help of Ken and slowly started to realize that life is about balance. The therapists needed time off and so did I. The weekends were the time to practice as well as relax, restore your energy, and try to find some peace.

Several times friends came to see me on weekends. Only Ken and Emily were allowed in the hospital, and not at the same time, so all these visits were outdoors. The summer was unusually hot. It always surprised me how hot it was, coming from the nice climate-controlled institution.

It was great to see our friends. It was a healthy dose of normality and a reminder of the love and support I had from many. I was a little nervous for visitors, at first. They would be seeing me with this huge incision on the back of my head and I was wheelchair bound, but these friends are like my family, and I know they love me.

Our good friends of close to thirty years, Lucy and her husband Rob, were the first to come. We had met in Grande Cache, becoming fast friends while raising our children together. Lucy welcomed us to her whole family. We have spent many special occasions at her family's farm, everyone making us feel like part of the family.

I was thrilled to see them, and they brought with them a container of fresh picked raspberries. It was the best gift as fresh food of any kind was limited in the hospital. Another friend, Joan, my cross-country ski partner, brought a special fuzzy blanket. It was so cozy. I kept it on my bed for the rest of my stay. One of my co-workers had become a close friend and she and her fiancé came several times to visit.

It's amazing how friends pop up from the most unexpected places. This incredible young woman came to work at the steel mill, while completing her Materials Engineering degree. We felt drawn to each other and as time went on our life circumstances firmly planted our friendship, growing into something I cherish. We had parallel situations with family estrangement and had both experienced a type of life-altering event. The roots of our friendship run deep. It has expanded to include her beautiful fiancé and they are forever woven into the fabric of our lives.

All these friends are like family to me. These are people who will always be an important part of life. I am so blessed. Not only these visitors, but I also had daily texts from both my sisters offering inspirational quotes and encouragement. I had regular phone calls with them as well as my parents. Other friends virtually checked in and Ken was receiving lots of support from our dear neighbours. My cloak of love and care was intact. My bouts of lugubriousness were short lived. How could they not be? I had to get better, I owed it to all these people who were always there for me.

One day I had a very special visitor. It was another hot day. It was Sunday, so I had no therapy. Ken had come that morning and helped me complete some of my exercises. After lunch Emily drove in. We would meet outside to adhere to COVID-19 mandates but also, she was bringing Arthur with her. My walking buddy. I missed that dog so much. Ken rolled me in my wheelchair to a grassy area in front of the hospital.

Soon Emily pulled up. I was so excited. So was Arthur. Being somewhere new, he was sniffing furiously. I called his name. His head popped up and he started pulling on his lead. Ken took over so Arthur's ninety pounds of exuberance wouldn't bowl me over. With his tail wagging like a windmill half his body joined me in my wheelchair and he started licking my face. We all got teary eyed.

It reaffirmed my resolve to walk. I would go for walks with Arthur again, no matter what! We had a lovely visit that seemed all too short, but I was tiring out and it was a long drive back for Ken and Emily. Emily took some photos and sent them to me. I treasured these and whenever I felt tired or sad, I would look at them, knowing what I was working towards.

HEALING INCISION

My head was healing nicely. The hospital had a therapy pool, and I was looking forward to going in the pool but first my stitches needed to come out. With the special continuous stitch the surgeon used, it was a different process for removing them. He had told me a doctor should do it. I relayed the information to the nursing staff, but they assured me this one nurse had the training to do it.

With trust in my nurses and apprehension in my heart, two of them came to remove my stitches. They had gauze pads, antiseptic cleaner and steri-strips ready. I asked them to take a before and after photo and they happily obliged, understanding my desire to document this event. My head was still quite numb so there was no pain, just a tugging feeling.

Before too long, it was done. One more step completed in my healing. Even my hair was starting to grow back. A few places were a little raw so they applied the steri-strips, and I would need to wait one more week before I could go swimming. I had the time, but I didn't like the idea of my hospital stay being measured in weeks.

The nursing staff were so kind and caring and offered lots of compassion. I depended on them and tried to convey my appreciation for their hard work. Even so, I didn't like how reliant on them I was. I had finally gotten approval to use the washroom independently. It was a rehabilitation hospital, so everything was set up for people with disabilities. This helped the patients be as independent as possible. I was becoming quite adept in maneuvering my wheelchair.

I should point out most of the staff wanted to do what was right for the patients and really cared. It was not just a job but a calling. As with any job, or even our calling, we all get tired, and we all need a break. These nurses got very few breaks. They were given a crazy schedule, seven days working for two off. Who came up with this insane timetable?

I remembered working at the steel mill. Some very aged employees had worked before using personal protective equipment was required. They were tired, they needed a break, and they had seen it all. They had gone through strikes and were sometimes not treated very well by those in power, subject to criticism. I approached these people with a smile, making it a personal goal to break through their fog of negativity. It usually worked.

Everyone has a story; everyone is going through something and perhaps life experiences have shaped their outlook. Everyone needs to be treated with kindness and respect and if I can help someone who maybe just needs a little more kindness, that's what I'm going to do. What does it cost me? Nothing. What might it do? Well, perhaps nothing but I need to believe that they will recognize that someone cares and maybe it will clear a little patch of their fog. As much as I relied on the nurses for my care, I tried to always ask them how they were and show compassion for their plight of being understaffed and overworked.

SHOWERS

One thing I still didn't like at all, as a patient, was shower time. First of all, with their busy schedule, they only offered showers twice a week. My mom shared stories of only weekly baths (in the same tub with the same water) when she was growing up, recounting her gratitude that she was the only girl in a family of four children, so she got her bath first. In our more modern world, I was used to more than twice weekly showers.

When the kindly staff helped someone to have a shower the process started in your room. You had to remove all your clothes there. You would transfer to a commode, or shower chair (sort of one and the same) and the staff would cover you with a large flannel blanket. They would then wheel you from your room to the shower room. There were three showers, separated by waterproof curtains. It brought back memories of when I used to teach aquafit at the pool.

The worst was watching other patients going for their showers. A commode is a waterproof wheelchair that has a large hole where your bottom is, convenient for people who needed help using the washroom. I was well acquainted with it. For showering, the nursing staff decently covered the naked patients with the large blanket, but often their butt was visible, below that big hole in the commode. Was mine showing like that? I didn't want to think about it.

Once in the shower, the staff set me up with the all-purpose soap/shampoo, washcloths, and the call button, for when I was done. At the University Hospital I needed help washing but now I could do it independently. Sitting on the commode/shower chair the staff gave me privacy, until I pressed the call button. I loved the feeling of the hot water, sluicing away several days' worth of living. I would have stayed longer but I knew the staff were busy and others were waiting for their prized shower time.

The staff wrapped me back up in a flannel blanket and wheeled me back to my room where I could get dressed. It was rejuvenating but also stressful. One evening I overheard my roommate talking to her adult daughter. They were talking about showers. My ears perked up. Every evening her daughter helped her shower. What was this? Maybe Ken could help me, and I wouldn't have to rely on the always so busy nursing staff.

First, I asked my nurse about it and sure enough Ken could help me. We just needed to ensure we didn't interfere with someone else's shower time. When Ken came to visit me, I told him about this revelation. Always there to support me, he heartily agreed. It was so much better. I got to go to the shower in my wheelchair and clothed, then transfer to a commode. Ken was there to help me. It felt so much more private and helped a lot with my sense of dignity although the nursing staff were very professional and compassionate. The best part was I could have more than two showers a week.

After helping me get setup, Ken stepped out so I could enjoy a longer shower. He then helped me get dressed in the shower area so there was no way I was showing off my backside to anyone. The nursing staff also let us in on another delightful secret. On the other side of the unit there was a single stall shower. One room, one shower. It was incredible. I absolutely loved it.

Ken was there for me, adhering to our wedding vows with a monumental amount of "In Sickness" dedication, always with a positive attitude. One shower time we had a good laugh over an unfortunate incident. Ken wanted to turn on the water before I was ready. The shower head was on a hose, leading from the tap. For someone who can't stand or move around much, this made showering much more feasible and pleasant. I asked him to wait but he turned it on, much to his chagrin. The shower head twisted on its cord and sprayed him, directly in the crotch and down one leg. It looked exactly as if he had had an "accident". I laughed out loud. Even Ken had to smile, a little. Ken said his pants remained wet until he got home and was able to change.

MOMENTS OF HUMOUR AND ADVENTURE

Finding moments of humour is crucial to healing. The rare moments of laughter infuse your body and soul with a renewed sense of energy and lighten your heart. We both worked hard to find bursts of our old selves within this strange, healing focused environment. We would go exploring around the hospital, inside and out. We discovered where the pool was located and a pediatric rehabilitation program. The bright colours and artwork were uplifting.

From my room on the fourth floor, I could see a courtyard. Ken and I decided to walk around the backside of the hospital to find it. Ken was pushing me in my wheelchair. It was too hard for me to maneuver any great distance with my right hand still regaining its strength and coordination. It was hard for Ken, with his shoulder injury. He had finally had soft tissue imaging done. It revealed that three of the four rotator cuff muscles were completely torn off. No wonder he still couldn't lift his arm out or up at all. No amount of physiotherapy was going to reattach those muscles. He was still waiting for an appointment with an orthopedic surgeon.

Thanks to COVID-19 and people who didn't believe our healthcare system was fragile, the staff were exhausted and overworked. It frustrated me beyond belief. When I was still in the University hospital, I overheard several conversations from visitors who believed the staff and government were lying to people about the severity of the pandemic. My pre-stroke self would have challenged their comments, but right then I just didn't have the energy. The healthcare workers remained professional, never wavering in their care. Firsthand I witnessed the full hospitals and saw that COVID-19 was still rampant.

Ken made the best out of his delayed injured shoulder treatment managing to push me in my wheelchair, one armed. We found the courtyard and had fun exploring with Ken taking photos of me after he pushed my wheelchair into a tunnel made for kids to play in. It was time to go back, and Ken suggested we try going back a different way, making a full circumference of the hospital. I said it was up to him and his arm as he had to navigate my wheelchair.

We embarked on this new path and soon found ourselves in a construction zone. Ken pushed on. We lost our sidewalk and had to go on the road. It was getting dicey but by this time it would be a long way to go back. We could see the main doors to the hospital, but it was a circuitous route to get to it. At one point, we were right beside the busy road in front of the hospital. With my vision challenges and being in a wheelchair, I just had to shut my eyes and hold on to the arm rests with an iron grip, hoping for the best.

We made it back, safe and sound. Ken was sweating, the exertion and stress taking its toll. We got to my room, and both had a laugh over our misadventure. I enjoyed retelling the tale during my therapy the next day. The therapist, a young, energetic and very knowledgeable woman told me about another possible venture. Across the busy road there was another, large hospital, offering full services, including an emergency department. She told me from the basement of this hospital there were tunnels that lead to the other hospital as well as a long-term care facility. They went right under the busy road. She said the other hospital had a really good food court and she would sometimes go there for lunch. I couldn't wait to tell Ken about it.

The next Saturday, after Ken helped me with my extra therapy exercises, we took the elevator to the basement. We looked around and found a sign that directed us to the other hospital. I maneuvered my wheelchair as much as possible, Ken taking over when I powered out. We followed the signs and saw a very long tunnel stretching before us. It was so long it looked like the hallways you see in horror movies that keep getting longer no matter how fast the survivor runs. To complete the effect, one of the overhead lights was flickering and there was a spot where water was dripping down.

When we were younger, we both loved a good horror movie. Every scary movie we ever watched flooded into our minds as we stared down the tunnel. We looked at each other and knew we were going. What an adventure! The tunnel echoed and we could hear the traffic rumbling overhead. Drip, drip went the water. Ken's footsteps reverberated off the walls. I started whispering the "Ja-Ja-Ja-Jason" from "Friday the 13th". It was fun but I don't think I would ever want to venture through that tunnel alone.

THE OTHER HOSPITAL

Once through the tunnel we needed to take another elevator to the main floor of the hospital. Since we were already inside, we avoided the COVID-19 guards. We started looking for the food court. There were parts of the hospital that reflected the agedness of the building and other parts that were vibrant and inviting. On the way to the food court, we saw signs indicating Healing Gardens. With memories of the peaceful gardens at the University Hospital we followed the signs.

These gardens were outdoors, on top of one of the roofs. It was complete with flowers, trees, water features, fish and smooth pathways throughout. It was beautiful. A little piece of paradise and respite within the confines of illness, medical emergencies, surgeries, and rehabilitation. We went there several more times during my hospital stay.

Eventually we found the food court. It was bright and had a fairly good variety even with some restaurants being closed due to the pandemic. They had my favourite, Tim Horton's. I LOVE their steeped tea. A steeped tea with 2 creams, there's nothing better. Ken got my tea and something for himself and we found a quiet spot to sit and enjoy it.

Yes, I was technically still in a hospital, but this was a different one and a much needed break from my own unit. As we sat, talking about my improvements and what our future was going to look like, I noticed something off in the distance. An elderly lady was walking, pushing her IV pole, tubes coming out of her left arm. She had bare feet and a flimsy hospital gown. The back of her gown was completely undone, exposing her nakedness underneath. She was shuffling, behind a staff person, trying to keep up. I assumed it was the elderly lady's support staff, who was about five feet ahead, looking at her phone. The staff looked back occasionally, then just kept walking, still looking at her phone. It bothers me to this day, although I've tried to write my own narrative that explains the situation and has a happy ending.

Anyone who's been hospitalized knows the loss of independence. You are bound by a different set of rules and schedules. It is a huge feat to care for so many sick people and it's overwhelming to think about the amount of organization it must take to meet everyone's medical, personal and nutritional needs. I believe they are trying their best. From my perspective and my volunteer work with Covenant Health, many patients in the hospital are sicker than in the past. Gone are the days of a week of care after an appendectomy. We were also experiencing an unprecedented time in this century with the ongoing world pandemic called COVID-19. As I've said before, what do you do when there is more need than capacity.

I was appreciative of the care I was receiving, despite all the ongoing challenges within healthcare. Ken and I explored the tunnels and what the other hospital had to offer several times. It was quite a distance for Ken to push me in my wheelchair. I was getting stronger and more adept at propelling myself, but I couldn't manage long distances. With Emily back home, she came to visit when she could.

One time after Emily and I had gone to the outdoor healing gardens of the other hospital, we took a side tunnel; one I hadn't gone through with Ken. It led to the Long-term care facility. On our way there was a row of hospital beds being stored. They were older than the one I had, reminiscent of the bed I had at the University Hospital. As we were walking by, we noticed one had a note taped to it. We bent over to read it - "Palliative Care. This bed works."

Emily and I leaned back and looked at each other. I'm sure it meant the mechanisms of the bed functioned but neither of us wanted to touch it, just in case. We had many moments, filled with adventure, fun, and good conversation. Emily was still managing her mental health and having her mom experience, yet another life-threatening situation presented challenges, I'm sure. I was proud of her tenacity to keep going.

We were all stumbling through, learning, and trying our best to support one another.

IMPROVING AMONGST CHALLENGES

I was improving, mostly in small incremental steps. Every relearned skill built upon another. Sometimes it came as a revelation but more often it was like a long forgotten memory reawakened. I was confident in my ability to transfer myself in and out of my wheelchair. I thought I should be able to walk but my legs just wouldn't cooperate with what my brain was telling it. I knew what they should do but it didn't happen. It was the strangest feeling. Brain injuries are filled with moments like this. You are thinking one thing, but your body does something completely different. It fills you with confusion because you know it's wrong but there's no path to the correct way. I guess that's what rehabilitation is all about; rebuilding new pathways to create a working map within your brain.

During all this hard work of reconstruction, I had to say goodbye to my roommate. We had become close in our few weeks together, but she had improved enough to return home. She shared her nervousness at this. She was excited to go home but was worried that the expectations of her old self would resurface, and she knew she could no longer do what she used to. It is one of the most frustrating things about having a brain injury. You can see your old self, but it's like a shadow, an apparition you can never really capture.

With my roommate leaving I expected I would be getting a new one. I remembered the assessors who came and saw me several weeks ago (had I really been here that long) telling me they had waiting lists. When I inquired about my new roommate, I was told I would be getting one later that day. Then to my surprise they told me it was a man.

A man? I was flabbergasted. At one of our meetings with Covenant Health, mixed gender rooms were an agenda item. We had a whole discussion on the appropriateness of mixed gender rooms. Now I was facing the exact prospect without any discussion. Would they have even prepared me had I not asked? I was beside myself and with my brain not processing things as quickly and my anxiety already heightened, I was upset.

There is already such a lack of privacy in a hospital and now I would be sharing my room with a man. The bathroom had sliding doors that did not come together all the way. The curtains, giving an illusion of privacy, were flimsy. Every sound filtered through the entire room. I felt so vulnerable and dependent and my dignity so fragile that this caused me a lot of apprehension. I was tired of this peripatetic hospital life and just wanted to be home in my own bed.

My protector and always my advocate, Ken saw my distress and tried what he could to alleviate my situation. He inquired about a private room, ensuring me his benefits program would cover most of the costs. This was all well and good, but all the private rooms were already being used as isolation rooms. Thanks again COVID-19! Short of discharging myself and going home, there was nothing we could do.

When Ken and I went for my usual exercise practice. I was still a little upset and the energy of my adrenalin flowed from my feelings and into my legs. Before long I had "walked" the farthest distance since my brain surgery. Even though I felt I was open-minded and used to working in a male dominated environment, I was uncomfortable. As I was listing off some of my concerns, my walking seemed to improve slightly. My dizziness and fatigue eventually caught up and Ken encouraged me to have a rest.

As I sat down, I gave a little sigh and let my negativity and worry over this male roommate go. As I've always said, the only thing we have control over is our choice. What was I going to choose here? I could be grumpy and complain or put on a smile and make the best of it. If you've read this far, you know what I chose. I recognized that this wasn't optimal, but I was grateful to receive excellent care and therapy from this specialized hospital. So, put on a smile and make the best of it, that's what I did.

As much as I wanted to be home, surrounded by my familiar environment and people who loved me, I knew the benefits I was gaining through the specialized rehabilitation I was receiving. I still couldn't walk or use my right hand properly and my vision was still coming together. I took a deep breath and dug a little deeper into my resolve to make the best out of this. Really, it wasn't that bad. My male roommate had no choice in having me, a woman, as a roommate either. We would both just have to make the best of it.

Like I said earlier, in life, we have no control. We are filled with hubris thinking of the control we impart over our daily lives but it's a mirage. When I think back to the control, I thought I had before my first stroke, I realize how arrogant I was. My first stroke taught me how small we are against the enormity of the forces surrounding us. Like people dealing with the aftermath of a Tsunami, or the person whose house was destroyed by a tornado whilst their neighbours went untouched. The examples are numerous and continuously remind us that we're not in control.

In my pre-stroke life, I thought I was in control. In fact, I was a control freak. I look back and I was a micromanager, even. I didn't think anyone could do it as well as me. Part of it was, and it's hard to admit, I felt if I was in control, I could keep those around me safe. A very early memory I have of an outing with my sisters and parents accentuates this. My Dad, the civil engineer and foundations specialist, wanted to collect some samples of Mica. Mica is a silicate mineral that is beautiful in its pearl like sheen and can peel off, almost paper thin.

There was an abundant deposit of Mica, but it was up a small rocky cliff. My Dad, ever the adventurer, quickly started climbing up the rocks. To me, the rock face loomed steeply, full of dangers. I reasoned if I climbed with him, it would be okay. In my little girl's brain, it made sense that if I were with him, he would need to keep me safe and through keeping me safe, he would be safe. Even then, I was a worrier. And I thought I could control things beyond anyone's command. Stroke was a very good teacher of how little control we really have.

There is something we can control completely. Our choice. The only thing we have control over are our choices and the decisions that follow. Bad things happen to good people, and like my mom and I like to say, nothing ever gets so bad it can't get worse. If you think about that seemingly pessimistic view, it is actually very heartening. If things can get worse, they are not so bad and if they are not so bad, they can get better. It's all dependent on you and your choices. It's a good paradigm shift towards a positive outcome; thanks mom!

Being melancholy and letting the circumstances determine your mood take far less effort. But that wouldn't help me get better any quicker or help me adjust to my new roommate. It would probably hinder it. However, it was a good fuel for working harder so I could return home as soon as possible, knowing I made the best of it. Life can throw all sorts of unexpected challenges at you. At the end of the day, all you can do is look back and see if you are proud of how you chose to respond. There are certainly days that I am not, but in reflection, I try to determine what I could have done and hopefully make a better choice next time.

"Yet, taught by time, my heart has learned to glow for another's good, and melt at other's woe." Homer

CHAPTER 10

CONGREGATE LIVING

I decided to welcome my new male roommate with a smile and kind words. This was what life was giving us and we needed to make the best out of it. I was filled with gratitude to be in this beautiful, professional rehabilitation hospital, getting first class treatment instead of lamenting I had a male roommate. Looking back, it really was minor, not something catastrophic.

My male roommate was getting used to the idea of being a stroke survivor. It is very overwhelming, knowing you've survived this deadly event but not unscathed. I felt for him when he had to call his wife to bring more pants. She kept asking why and finally he had to tell her it was because he had peed his pants, again. He was a proud man, and I knew how difficult it must have been for him to say this.

After a stroke, you know you are different, just trying to survive each day, finding normality within your new normal. It's a long road and I considered myself lucky to have travelled so far on it already because of my first strokes. And for me it was a long journey. I was in so much denial, I was going back to work come hell or high water, I wouldn't even use the word stroke. When I looked into the faces of new stroke survivors, I saw a mirror image of what I experienced; the disbelief, the denial, the questions, the overlying uncertainty of "Who am I now?"

Part of the rehabilitation offered was sessions with a neuropsychologist. A neuropsychologist is a psychologist who specializes in understanding the relationship between the physical brain and behavior. This one was a very kind and intelligent young woman. I met with her initially to see if I was adjusting well to being a stroke survivor. I told her, truthfully, although it was a difficult road, I considered myself very fortunate because I had been travelling this road for a while. I knew what to expect and I knew I was lucky. I had lost a lot, more than once, but I was still here and despite some differences, I was mostly still me.

I had gone through the initial shock of what it meant to be a stroke survivor the first time. For my co-patients I could see the shock, disbelief, the grieving in their eyes, in their loved one's eyes. The unanswered question, "How could this happen to me?" I would listen to their stories; they were healthy, there was no warning, how could this happen, they would have to sell their house, they were leaving a sick spouse at home alone. So much hurt, need, and grieving. Some were like soldiers, returning from battle, a shell-shocked look about them. They had survived but not intact.

I've mentioned this before, but it is such a unique experience, I'll write a little more about it. The bond created between patients is beyond words. Usually when you meet someone for the first time, it might be at a party, a work conference, school, generally when you're out and about. At those times you are usually dressed for whatever occasion it might be and on your best behaviour. We present our best, practiced outside self for everyone to see, trying to make a good first impression. Relationships grow from there and as we build trust, we let people see beneath the glossy surface into who we really are.

When I met other patients at the hospital, we were all at different levels of our worst. That was our starting point. There were no polished packages around our true selves, we were all just trying to survive and navigate the roller coaster ride. There was relief in that. We could just be our damaged selves and accept each other where we were on the ride. More importantly, we understood and saw the beauty reflecting into us, knowing we were warriors, each of us fighting our own battle yet finding reassurance in each other's company.

I tried to talk to people, offering my words, hoping they provided just a smidgen of a balm for the invisible wounds caused by stroke. I told them we were in an exclusive club, stroke survivors. We would get through. If it was appropriate, I offered the advice of that wise charge nurse who spoke with me while I was in the special care unit at St. Mary's hospital all those years ago.

Holding my hand gently she told me, "Having a stroke is akin to a loss, you've lost a part of yourself. Give yourself time to grieve, to rest. Stroke is a life-altering event so give yourself a break. One step, one day at a time. Recovery will happen for the rest of your life."

This hit the proverbial nail on the head for me. My life was turned upside down, I needed to give myself time to grieve. I needed to be open to what the roller coaster ride of life presented and be open to the possibilities and new opportunities created by stroke. It certainly wasn't what I had planned but perhaps it is what was meant to be. This took me almost four years to discover and come to terms with.

Then I had another stroke. I'm not minimizing what I was going through this time, but having had a stroke previously was an advantage. I didn't need to grieve my loss of work. I had already lost and relearned so many of my previous abilities. I had firm belief I would regain most again.

WHAT'S IMPORTANT

I've learned my lessons and figured out what was important in life; waking up each morning, greeting a new sunrise, letting family and those close to me know how much I love them, how much I appreciate them. I discovered joy in seeing the birds at our feeder instead of making my quota at work. I had had four years to get used to what it meant to be a stroke survivor, and it gave me an edge in dealing with this latest one. I could recognize that some of the other patients were still in the first stage. It's a journey and you have to go through each part at your own speed. Last time I tried to rush it using denial and busyness and I feel my family suffered for it.

I have an amazing support network, people who truly care for me. I had already been through the devastation of losing my career and I knew what it took to get lost skills back. It was a bumpy road, but I would be okay, and I told the neuropsychologist so. She believed me but I still needed to go through a process to determine any lost cognitive skills. Her assistant would administer several tests for a variety of cerebral processes, including memory, patterns, math, language, reasoning, and it seemed like a ton of others. It would take three, one-hour sessions to complete them all. I was always a games aficionado with a competitive streak! Challenge accepted!

The tests certainly challenged me. I tried so hard and always needed a nap after these sessions. We did multiple memory tests, reasoning tests, math, language and on and on. The neuropsychologist scheduled another meeting once I was done all the testing to inform me of my results. I was nervous, so tentative was my grasp on how much I had changed. I felt mostly like me, but was I really? I say this seriously, not tongue in cheek, brain injuries really mess with your mind.

We had a good session, and I shared my struggles and acceptance of my male roommate and that generally I was doing okay. She moved onto the results. On the whole, I had pretty normal results for someone my age. Phew! In a few areas, I did better than average and these included memory and patterns. Yahoo! I really think music and bass playing lent a hand in improving those skills.

Rehabilitation continued daily as well as my extra practice. Soon I was able to graduate to a four-wheeled walker. The four-wheeled walker needed more balance and strength to operate. I was thrilled to now be able to manage one. Just like all my other mobility equipment, I was given one, with my name on it, to keep in my room and use throughout my stay. I still had my wheelchair but was trying to rely mostly on my new walker.

I had been relearning so many balance and mobility skills and Ken and I continued the extra therapy every evening. One day my therapist strapped me into a harness, and I walked up and down the hallway in the harness, attached to a ceiling track. It felt good to walk upright. Although I was weaving about and wobbly, I loved the exercise without fear of falling. The weight on my right foot helped to control my stride.

Other exercises worked on a variety of skills. One exercise challenged my balance, standing and my vision, all in one. With a transfer belt on and the therapist ready to steady me, I would stand in front of a large computer screen. I mean really large, almost as tall as me and wider than I could stretch my arms. The therapist could access multiple "games" designed to help with vision and balance. They certainly worked on mine.

One exercise consisted of a turning wheel with letters scattered all around. A letter would turn a different colour and I would need to touch it in a predetermined amount of time. Another game had numbers moving from side to side, all mixed up and I would have to look around and locate them sequentially and touch them before they reached the end of the screen. I found these exercises fun, dizzying and something different that targeted so many of the skills I was trying to regain. I was in this hospital to improve, and I might as well have a good time doing it.

RECREATION

My motivation was such that I signed up for all the extra recreational activities I could. On Thursday afternoons I joined a Wii bowling group. The therapist was extremely helpful, setting us up and busy ensuring our remotes were working. We were all in wheelchairs and I was impressed how well we could play from a sitting position. I also joined an art class.

Once a week, I would make my way in my wheelchair, getting lost just about every time, to the art room. It would have been an Art Teacher's dream room. It was open, roomy, had art project tables and every supply you could think of. The therapist assistant led us through a process for painting with water colour pencils. I'm not much of an artist but had fun trying it out. My male roommate joined this class as well and I was impressed with his artistic ability. I think he was too, saying he had never painted before.

We were making things work, in our room. We chatted through the thin curtain, getting to know each other. We got to know more than we wanted but had an unspoken agreement to keep those things private. One day, though, I was having a rest in my bed and my roommate was being helped in the washroom. He had finished when the healthcare aide started exclaiming, surprisedly, he shouldn't do that. Being able to hear absolutely everything, I realized my roommate decided to wash his hands in the toilet. "It's the same water that comes out of the tap!" he told the aide. He tried to convince me of the cleanliness of toilet water later, knowing I heard the exchange. Each to their own but I continued to use the sink to wash up.

He wasn't the tidiest, and his deficits added to the problem. The cleaners only came in once a day. I mentioned the state of our washroom to one of my aides. Her solution was to bring me a tub of disinfecting wipes and latex gloves. What do you do? Sitting in my wheelchair, I cleaned up the washroom when I needed to.

My roommate was a bit of a redneck if I could be so bold as to use that term. He reminded me of some of the steelworkers from the mill. Good people, solid values, and a little old fashioned. He was the one who pointed out that the obscure patterns on our curtains were reminders of nature - leaves, snails, birds, and seashells. I appreciated his curtain comparison. He was a Jehovah's Witness. I saw his church come together, through Zoom, to support him through his stroke and recovery. He never pushed me except to offer me a place at one of his virtual meetings after I helped him join in when he was having problems with the passcode.

Overall, it was okay except at nighttime. He slept a lot during the day. I could hear him snoring contentedly many times in between his therapy sessions. At night he would listen to the radio. I asked him to use headphones. He had to use the washroom many times during the night and needed nursing staff assistance. It was extremely disruptive. And he would eat. It seemed everything he ate was wrapped in a crinkly plastic he spent minutes taking off. Then all the food was crunchy. Munch, munch, munch! One time I woke myself up, yelling "Shut Up!" in my sleep, his noisiness entering into my dreams. My roommate was again listening to the radio. I hope my sleep muddled brain didn't allow me to actually form the words. He did shut off the radio after that though.

Sleeping in a hospital is arduous enough without a night owl for a roommate. I spoke to one of my nurses about it, telling her how tired I was and that my headaches were getting worse. I had visions of her privately mentioning to him to please be quiet during the night. I had tried but really wasn't successful. I wasn't as forthcoming as I should have been, being too worried about offending him. That's when an archaic practice the hospital engaged in came back to bite me, hard.

SHIFT CHANGE

Every shift change, the entirety of both units would go from room to room. At the doorway of each the head nurse would do an update on the patients living there. They would loudly comment on sleeping, eating, therapy and bowel movements. They shared this information in front of us, about us but did not include us. As much as my care was kind and compassionate, this practice made me feel like an animal in the zoo.

The morning after I had mentioned my sleeping problems and my roommate, they stood by our doorway, my roommate and I each in our respective beds, and loudly stated how C. Holubec-Jackson complained she was not sleeping well because her roommate was too noisy. After finishing the update, they left, nothing else. I was mortified. So was my roommate. I apologized to him but saw this as an opportunity. Taking a deep breath, I asked if he could try not to eat during the night and always use headphones if he wanted to listen to the radio.

Living with another person who is a stranger, you learn a lot. You learn to accept each other's idiosyncrasies. You even learn to be more of an advocate for yourself, saying what needs to be said, while maintaining compassion for the circumstances that led us to being hospitalized. You learn tolerance and even form a friendship through your shared trauma. We were in this together and we both recognized we needed to make this work.

We tried hard and it did work. I also became a little sly in that whenever I noticed him napping during the day, I would do something noisy to wake him up. He slept better those nights and so did I. An incident did occur to disrupt our sleep and I still laugh about it today. It was about 11:30 at night. We were both sleeping when a cell phone started ringing. It rang and rang and then stopped. I knew it wasn't mine. Then it started again. I called out from my bed, "Answer your phone!" He told me it wasn't his, it was mine. It stopped but almost immediately started again. We were both wide awake by now.

Maybe one of the nursing staff left their phone in our room? I was able to transfer myself into my wheelchair, so I offered to go look. I couldn't find any phone anywhere. It stopped and started again. I asked him to call the nurse, maybe it was in his bag. The nurse came and discovered his wife had left her phone in the drawer of his bedside table. The nurse handed it to him and left. My roommate stated his son was probably trying to figure out where her phone was.

Now we could sleep. My roommate was still rummaging around, trying to make sense of the two phones he now held in his hands, his own and his wife's. He called his wife's phone, using his. I heard it ringing and I heard the wife's phone go to voice mail. I was cranky, sleepy, and irritated by this late-night disturbance but what happened next had me laughing. When the voice mail went to messaging, my roommate left his wife a very stern one. "You left your phone here, I guess you can pick it up later. And STOP calling here! People are trying to sleep!" He hung up while I lay giggling to myself.

Such is hospital life and congregate living. Patients came and went from our unit and soon a spot became available in a male room and my roommate was moving. I would be getting a new roommate, a female. As much as we were making the best of our situation, I was elated. My new roommate arrived, with her husband. We had many similarities in our situation as well as a lot of differences.

ANOTHER NEW ROOMMATE

We were similar in age and had lots of support from our husbands. Her stroke was caused by a brain bleed too; an aneurysm four months previous. She had to have emergency brain surgery to manage it. She had a different surgeon than mine. After surgery she was left with a lot more challenges than me. She had spent several weeks in the hospital and was then transferred to long-term care, waiting to come to this rehabilitation hospital. Three months she had been waiting. I didn't understand why.

Her husband was beside himself trying to cope with the changes stroke caused in his wife as well as advocate for her rehabilitation care. Ken spent some time talking with him as did I. For some reason, and I think it has to do with the level of disability they could manage, the hospital felt they were not able to provide her with adequate therapy. Besides personal care difficulties, his wife had trouble speaking, her speech being impacted causing something called aphasia.

Aphasia is a language disorder caused by damage in a specific area of the brain that controls language expression and comprehension. Aphasia leaves a person unable to communicate effectively with others. She could form words but often her words weren't connected to what she was trying to say. I've heard other people describe this as "word salad", saying a jumble of words strung together. I could see her frustration. She was aware her words weren't what she wanted to say. I spent time talking with her and despite her aphasia and jumbled words, she communicated very well. She had great family support between her husband and her sister.

My new roommate touched me in a way that reached my soul. I realized anew how lucky I was and thanked God for it. I believe bad things happen to all of us, it's just the way it is. I also believe that God had a hand in softening my blows as much as possible. My latest hemorrhage was a more significant bleed, but it bled into my ventricle instead of destroying even more brain tissue. It pushed out the malformation, so the surgeon felt confident to operate. My operation was a success. Even with my new deficits, I knew I would get those skills back, but most importantly I was still me! And my cloak of care from so many was still wrapped around, ensuring I had love and support every step of the way. I will never forget how blessed I am.

One thing all these different roommates taught me was that everyone, each one of us, has a story. Our lives are an accumulation of our life experiences. A tale forged in memories made, challenges met, momentous moments. Memories that bring smiles to our faces. Some that will forever hold a special place in our hearts, darker moments, that we leave locked in a box, only to be let out when we are strong enough to let them ruminate in our minds.

Every person is made of these events that made them what they are when they entered into our lives. Stroke shaped the people I met, the reason we found ourselves as comrades. Our relationships feel like they have been in existence forever because of their intensity and the magnitude of shared emotions but they are actually very fleeting.

GOING SWIMMING

Soon my incision had healed enough that the doctor felt I could try swimming. I was excited. I had always loved swimming, had taught swimming lessons, coached competitive swimming, taught aquafit, even participated in a Triathlon. When I was young, I had read "The Little Mermaid". I couldn't understand why the mermaid wanted legs and to live on land. I wanted a tail and go live under the sea! I often had dreams that I was plunged into the ocean and unable to reach the surface. Right at the moment I thought I would drown - I remembered I could breathe underwater. I started breathing and exploring. I loved those dreams and wished I really could breathe underwater. I haven't had that dream in a while.

The Recreation Therapy Assistant brought me to the swimming pool. It was a small therapy pool with a zero-depth entrance and railings, perfect for people with mobility challenges. Wearing a transfer belt, the lifeguard helped me into the water. The water was warm, like a soothing bath. Much better than my memories of 6:30 AM Aquafit in a chilly competition pool. Once I was chest deep, the lifeguard let go of the transfer belt. I was standing by myself. What a feeling. After so much time dependent on my wheelchair or walker or someone else, I was standing independently. It was a beautiful moment.

I walked back and forth in the pool, the warm water supporting me, buoying my arms and legs, bearing the brunt of my weight. My dreams of living underwater flooded back. Here I felt like I was the master of my own body. I had escaped the weight of gravity and could be independent. It was beautiful.

The lifeguard was right there to help me, if needed. I was walking, she mentioned she knew me and asked if I remembered her. I took a closer look. She was familiar but I couldn't place where I knew her from. She told me she was a friend of Kaylyn's, my still estranged eldest daughter. They had gone to university together. She recalled when she and Kaylyn had taken an extra-curricular course in making and racing on an ice luge.

That I remembered. Kaylyn had always loved the cold, and winter sports. On top of all her courses, she had been working hard to take part in this extracurricular ice luge course. When the luge was finished the professor held a fun race for all the students. Spectators were invited. The high for the day was -18*c with a slight wind. It was cold! I took time off work to come and watch. Bundled up, I walked partway up the hill and took pictures of Kaylyn and others racing down the luge course at breakneck speeds. I was the only spectator to come and watch the culmination of all their hard work.

Now I could place this supportive, kind lifeguard. She had even been to our house once. She asked about Kaylyn, and I was evasive, saying the little I knew while being vague about our relationship. I had enough on my plate and didn't want to go into any details about Kaylyn distancing herself from our family. The swimming was over, all too soon. It had been wonderful, but I was tired. Back in my room, I laid down and rested, waiting for Ken to come after he was done work.

"Grief never gets any smaller, so you have to get bigger around it."
J. Ridgeway, *Locke & Key*

CHAPTER 11

TOO LONG A PATIENT

The next time Emily came to visit I told her about meeting the lifeguard who knew Kaylyn. Emily told me, almost awkwardly, that Kaylyn had reached out to her. They had been chatting over text. Emily was elated to have her big sister back in her life. She also thought Kaylyn wanted to find out how I was doing. Did she still care? Why didn't she just text or call me. The familiar sadness threatened to overwhelm me again, but I just didn't have the capacity to manage anything more. I settled on hoping this reunion between Emily and Kaylyn would lead to her coming back to our family. I could never have predicted how spectacularly it would fail.

Another person who was in contact with Kaylyn came for an outdoor visit. It was the young neuroscientist who now had his PhD, who was our inspiration for a brainy superhero, Ty the Neuro Guy. He lived in Calgary but was in Edmonton for collaboration as he was starting his own neuroscience-based business. It was so good to see him, he had a deeper understanding of what my brain had been through and was always very compassionate.

We had a wonderful visit, reminiscing about his and Kaylyn's high school days and talking about his venture. He was and is very ambitious. I knew he would do well. We were proud of him, and it melted my heart when he told us he thought of us as his second set of parents. We assumed he was staying with his parents and Ken offered him a ride home. Almost sheepishly, he told us he was staying with Kaylyn, who lived right in Edmonton. I barely held it together. How many times can your heart break?

We hugged and I thanked him for taking the time to come visit me. Ken took me back to my room. We talked about the lovely visit but decided not to bring up the fact Ty was staying with Kaylyn. What more could we say? I think she still loves me. I think she cares. I hold onto that.

That night, as I was getting ready for bed, there was a terrific thunderstorm. I had a view of the city, towards the football stadium. It was lit up with colour changing lights every night. This night the whole sky was illuminated with flashes of lightening, so intense I could see whole forks streaking through the sky. The thunder penetrated the thick walls overpowering the hum of the continuous fans within the hospital. It was an incredible show of the magnificent power of nature. It seemed one streak of lightning hit the ground right by the stadium, the lights around it went dark. I felt that important reconnection to nature surface. I sat on my bed watching, the storm purging itself of its' intensity. I fell asleep as an occasional low rumble continued throughout the night.

The next morning, I rose to a beautiful sunny sky, with only whisps of fluffy white clouds dotted here and there. The roof just beyond was turned into a water feature, huge puddles almost covering it completely. The light was just right, and it looked almost like a tropical location with pools below me. I took a few photos and got ready for the day.

STARTING THE DAY AND NEW STAFF

Usually, I tried to be dressed before the nursing staff came in to see how my night was and take my vital signs. Looking out my window and taking photos put me behind and the nurse came in with a new trainee. She was a young, energetic healthcare aide and I was happy to see more staff joining as I knew how hard everyone there worked.

After the initial good mornings, I tried to talk with her as she took my vitals, but I could tell she was nervous and looked to her mentor for a lot of direction. They chatted back and forth a lot, her mentor helping my roommate. I wasn't really listening, but I heard her ask, "Should I help her get dressed?" The mentor replied, "You can look at her chart." I perked up as she started looking at my chart. Was I the "her" they were talking about? I looked up from my lower position in the wheelchair, and asked if they were talking about me? She sheepishly nodded her head, yes. "I'm verbal, we were just talking. You can just ask me if I need help?"

Maybe I was a little curt, but I was vexed at the thoughtlessness. This was yet another example of why the work I was doing with Covenant Health was so important. Staff needed reminding that patients and their families should be valued members of their own healthcare team. This new staff person didn't even consider asking me what I needed, after talking to me just moments before. I don't think she was unkind or uncaring, I feel she just didn't think. I was the patient, the job, not an individual. This is where the promotion of patient engagement as the norm not the exception is vital to develop as a culture within healthcare.

On the heels of this was another frustrating event. I guess I was improving enough to start noticing my lack of independence and decision making. I just wanted to be home. Every night I was still getting my injection in my stomach for the blood thinner. Every time I asked about it, they told me as long as I was in a wheelchair, I needed it.

But I wasn't using my wheelchair as often. Continued practice and doing my exercises were paying off. I was mastering using my four-wheeled walker. I was even able to go to my therapy sessions using my walker instead of the wheelchair. That was a huge improvement. I really didn't want to be on the injection anymore. My stomach was constantly bruised from the needle. It seemed I missed the morning visits from the travelling doctor and nurse practitioner as I was in therapy, and my messages to them from my nurse didn't seem to get through.

One Sunday morning, I was sitting in my bed finishing breakfast, when one of the doctors came in. He peeked around my curtain and asked how I was doing. Here was my chance! I told how much I felt I was improving. I launched into my desire to stop having the needle every night. He casually told me my physiotherapist was the one to order the stop of this medication. He said this while leaving, not even looking at me.

My physiotherapist had the power to change my medication? This was news to me and to her. She said she would pass on a message about my improvement. She felt I was walking quite a bit and had improved immensely but it wasn't for her to decide. After several more days, I still didn't have any follow-up or answers. That night I told my nurse this would be the last night I would receive the injection. Tomorrow night I would refuse the medication because I felt no one was listening to me and I didn't think I needed it anymore.

I'm not a problem patient, I don't think. If someone gave me a good explanation for continuing the medication, I would have taken it, no problem. It was like when they introduced the medication, over a month ago now, once it was explained it made sense. The explanation they were giving me now, that I needed to walk more, didn't make sense. I was walking, albeit with help, but I was mobile.

TIRED OF HOSPITAL LIFE

Times like this I had a growing feeling of being a job, losing my humanity in the realm of being just another chore. Most staff were amazing, but a few reinforced the feeling being a job. I'm sure they were tired or burnt out. I was just another task on their list of things to do. One nurse tried to trick me by grabbing one of my Kleenexes to disinfect my stomach before she jabbed me with a needle since she forgot an alcohol swab. Maybe I should have said something, but I didn't. I remember a friend of ours who was a vice-principle, talking about "red flag parents", the ones who were always complaining. I didn't want to be a "red flag patient" and I was worried my feelings were coloured by my own attitude. I'm sure a lot of my anxiety was being projected into their innocuous behaviour, lacing it with my own insecurities.

Never, in my wildest dreams, did I imagine being away from home so long. It was beyond frustrating. My mind was intact, but my body wasn't cooperating. I always tried to put on a smile, asked others how they were, wished them a good day but sometimes it wore on me. I tried making the choice to be positive but occasionally that would slip. Ken would see the real struggles, the frustrations, the sadness.

I realized I was at an impasse. Was the stress of being a patient out-weighing the benefits I was receiving from therapy? Were all these little incidents that seemed cumulative signs telling me it was time? Or were these teachers, helping me to get over any hubris and accept the help. I may not need all of it, but I definitely need most of it. I needed to get rid of my attitude and welcome their care with open arms and kindness, while advocating for patients everywhere instead of being upset.

The next morning the nursing staff informed me they had spoken to the doctor, and he decided I didn't need the blood thinner injection anymore.

Yay! A small victory of self-advocacy. It was hard telling the nursing staff I would refuse the medication. It's so much easier just to do what you're told and not cause any waves. I had talked it over with Ken before and he helped me find the courage to talk to them, leading to the change in my medication. I was also starting to feel better and find a little more independence even within my dependent, congregate living situation.

MY EYES

One area that was not showing as much improvement were my eyes. My occupational therapist had hoped for more improvement, so she booked me an appointment at the Alberta Eye Health Clinic to check it out. It was for the next day and unfortunately Ken already had work meetings planned. He couldn't have driven me but would have come along. My therapist had booked me a special, wheelchair accessible taxi to take me to the appointment. She told me they used this one all the time and he knew his way around the hospital and the different clinics patients went to for appointments.

I was nervous. This would be the first time in weeks, except for the ambulance ride, I would be leaving the hospital. Again, I would be without Ken. They say there is no courage without fear, so I must have been very brave that day. Kelly's Taxi service came right to my unit to pick me up. He seemed like a very nice man, all business and efficient. I asked him if his name was Kelly, expecting it not to be, and was surprised it was. It's like going to Luigi's Pizza, you don't expect the employee's to be named Luigi. I guess it was his own business and he was the sole employee.

He loaded me into the back of his accessible van. He strapped down the wheelchair and off we went. I had mixed reactions. It was great to be out, and I realized we were really close to a nice mall I had gone shopping to years ago with Kaylyn. But being in a wheelchair in the back of a mini van was quite bumpy and jumpy. Edmonton is not known for smooth roads, and it felt like we hit every pothole.

He took me to the eye clinic; a small office and it seemed the area was a little rough. He parked in the back alley. He went to the door, texted a number and the staff came and opened it. He pushed me in, then told me the office would call once I was done and he'd pick me up. It felt a little like one of those crime movies where one of the underlings was meeting to represent the big boss. Maybe I watch too many movies.

Everyone at the clinic was very nice but they seemed surprised at my arrival. One assistance asked what they could do for me today. Hadn't the therapist called and arranged all this? They were also not set up for someone in a wheelchair. It was very awkward, for all of us. Before I let any of my feelings of insecurity disable me further, I sat up straighter in my chair and tried to answer their questions. They still seemed confused, but the optometrist took me for an exam.

It felt like he didn't have much experience with stroke survivors or brain injuries. Fortunately, I did. I knew some of the words to describe my condition and he asked what I needed from him. I didn't know. I thought he would have an idea of something that could help. I gave him the paperwork from the therapist and described my condition, using words like diplopia and nystagmus which I had learned; Diplopia means double vision, and nystagmus is involuntary movement of your eyes.

He wrote down these things and had nothing further to offer. What was the point of this visit? The therapist had praised the accolades of the clinic. I learned later that there is another Alberta Eye Clinic that is called the Eye Institute of Alberta which is in the Royal Alexandra Hospital. The same hospital we took the tunnels to visit. It's a first-class eye health clinic with ophthalmologists, who have different specialties. On my first outpatient visit with my neurosurgeon he referred to me this clinic to see a neuro-ophthalmologist. Maybe Kelly's Taxi took me to the wrong clinic, that's why they were surprised to see me. I can laugh about it now although at the time it caused me quite a bit of stress.

I WANT TO GO HOME

I was getting impatient of being a patient. I was improving and just wanted to have some of my independence back. I was getting better at managing my four wheeled walker, which would make it easier at home. When our friends came for another outdoor visit, I was able to meet them outside, using only my walker. In the evenings Ken was also helping me walk with just my pole. I was wobbly and needed help, but I could do it. Again, I told Ken when I left, I would walk out, just using the pole. We practiced stairs too as we live in a two-story house. I was very self-motivated and would continue my exercises on my own.

It had been over five weeks of being in a hospital and I was more than ready to go home. I talked to my therapists, and they agreed, if I had enough help at home. They started preparing me for home life. The physiotherapist started doing testing for balance and if I could get up from the floor, imitating having fallen. She also found a place in Wetaskiwin where we could borrow a walker, free of charge.

The hospital had several mini kitchens and the occupational therapist arranged for me to practice some cooking skills. Using a knife, walking around the kitchen, using the stove were all important skills. I was so nervous the first time I tried. My hand was shaky, and my balance was unsteady as I moved around, using the counter for balance and support. It felt so good to be cooking again. I love cooking and baking, even though I really can't taste much of it. It's so satisfying creating something for others to enjoy. Food brings people together. I missed it and was proud of my chocolate chip oatmeal cookies. I shared them around the unit, smiling from ear to ear.

Ken was thrilled. He missed my food too. He finished off the cookies, managing to save one to take home to Emily. We made plans for my return home in the next week. He had ordered a shower chair for me. Standing to shower takes a lot of balance, something I was still working on. Having the shower chair would make things easier and safer. He also contacted the Medi-Lend and got a walker for me to use, free, for three months. Things were coming together, and I was elated.

The last exercise my therapist wanted to practice was walking outside with my four wheeled walker. I had done some, but now she wanted me to walk on the sidewalk and cross the road. I was a little nervous. This was a busy road, with traffic lights and cross walks. It was the same busy road Ken, and I ended up beside when we had our adventure through the construction zone when I was still in my wheelchair. It surprised me how a simple thing like crossing the road, using my walker, made me so nervous.

Pushing myself to move faster, we made it, no problem. I didn't like the vehicles whooshing past me, so close. With someone with sensory challenges and vision issues, maybe it's understandable. I needed to be less critical of myself. I think we're often our own worst critic.

GETTING READY TO GO HOME

Ken started taking some of my stuff home so it wouldn't be so much the day I left. There were a few loads. Between my bass, my computer, clothes, personal supplies, books, it added up. Finally, the day before I was to leave, I had just the bare minimum in my room, my home away from home. I wanted to be in my real home so badly, but I would miss the new friends I had made. Also, I wanted to show my appreciation to the nursing staff for all they did for me.

Ken and I talked, and he would make a gift basket for the unit. He would put in lots of individually wrapped snacks and other little things that would hopefully offer things for a quick break during their busy shifts. We also included some of our Glia Girl books. It was all about stroke and what better place to start promoting it than a specialized stroke rehabilitation hospital unit. I gave a copy to my therapists and my stroke doctor. They all seemed very appreciative. I gave a copy of the book to some of the friends I had made too.

There was such a feeling of support and love between all the patients. We were all there for the same reason. We understood, like no one else could, what it's like to recover from a stroke. We praised each other on our successes and cried together when we had setbacks. We knew the challenges of sleeping in a hospital and the lack of privacy. We laughed about the short mealtime delivery and looked away when someone was be taken to the shower, butt sticking out. They were my brethren, and I would miss them.

I was so grateful to be able to go home. Ken and I became good friends with one other patient and her husband. The husband appreciated talking to Ken. Like Ken, he came to the hospital every day. He had his own health issues and his wife had more significant challenges than me. To manage her needs she would end up going to an assisted care facility. Saying goodbye to them was hard. We tried to instill as much hope and love as possible into our words. We still keep in touch, and her husband still visits her every day.

The connections I've made at the hospital are truly a blessing. These people are more than just other patients, they are friends. We've cried and celebrated together. We know things about each other that most people never know about their friends. There is a bond stronger than steel, forged by our shared experiences with stroke. The staff will be forever remembered, for all the care, the compassion, the jokes, the encouragement, just knowing they are always there, watching out for us, keeping us safe and as healthy as possible. I never thought it would affect me like this. That I would grow so attached.

I spent most of the summer in the hospital. It's been so long since I've slept in my bed, seen our home, our garden. I can't help feeling a sense of wonder. Sometimes it feels like this whole experience has just been a dream, did this really happen to me? It did, and I'm coming home. I'm so grateful for how far I've come. I still have a way to go but that's okay. I'll get there. I appreciate every little thing. I've seen how it could have been. I know how lucky I am.

My last night, I fell asleep, listening to the gentle breathing of my roommate. I was anxious to go home but a little nervous too. In the hospital, I had very few decisions to make. My days were laid out and always included ample time for breaks. I know myself and know how hard it is for me to rest when other things are going on. My newest normal also didn't like making decisions and found too many things going on stressful. I had shared my apprehensions with Ken, and I knew he would help me through yet another transition.

I had several good things happening once I got home to look forward to. Kevin and Alix would be visiting soon, after giving me a few days to adjust to home life. I hadn't seen Kevin since that brief visit shortly after my surgery and it had been over a year since I'd seen Alix, due to COVID-19 and travel restrictions. Then on the heels of their visit my sister, Cami would come.

Cami lived in Niagara Falls. We usually visited at least once a year, but again COVID-19 delayed things. I didn't expect her to come until later. My parents were supposed to come but increasing COVID-19 cases had them worried. Our premier had changed masking and social gathering restrictions just before my surgery, announcing that Alberta was "Open for Summer". The fast-climbing cases, hospitalizations and deaths was indicative of what a poor decision that was. With both my parents being in their eighties, they made the hard decision not to come, even though it had been years since we had seen each other because of COVID-19. Luckily Cami's visit would fill the void.

LAST HOSPITAL DAY

I woke up my usual early and noticed the sun was just starting to rise. The sun rises early in Alberta in the summer and was usually already in my eyes when I woke up. The days were starting to get shorter. Fall was just around the corner. I'd spent almost a whole season in the hospital.

I did my usual morning ablutions, then packed up the last of my personal items so I'd be ready to go home at the end of the day. My feelings were still dichotomous. On one hand I was so excited to go home, I'd more than enough of hospital life. On the other, I was nervous, would I manage alright?

Regardless of my divisive feelings, there was no way I was staying another night. I took a deep breath and waiting for the nursing staff to take their morning vitals check. Everything was good and all the staff who came were so kind and full of positive comments and well wishes for my departure. Many flouted the COVID-19 protocols and gave me a hug! Even though there had been some challenges, on the whole my care had been supreme. I will be forever grateful for how much I received in care and rehabilitation during my stay. I know how lucky I am to be in a country that offers services like this. And we didn't have to pay anything out of pocket.

Our healthcare system is worldclass. I know there are lots of problems and COVID-19 has surely tested it but imagine if I had been somewhere without a public healthcare system. Would I have even been able to afford the operation? I have read many Twitter posts from people in other countries who did not have access, opportunity, or funds to receive the kind of medical care and rehabilitation I had.

So, yes, I am very grateful, and I do not take for granted what I just received. I was sure to extend my heartfelt thanks to everyone I saw that day. I profusely thanked all my therapists and gave them a copy of the Glia Girl book. So many times, my thank you's seemed so small for the monumental support I received. They wanted me to come for a few outpatient visits, but it was a long drive, and I wasn't sure how I would manage it. Ken was going to try and organize something with the nearby hospital that offered me home rehabilitation after my first stroke, the Stroke – Early Supported Discharge program. They had given me such amazing care and rehab then as well as compassionate understanding as I tried to make sense of my new normal.

The day went by quickly and soon Ken was there to pick me up. He took my last bags to the car and then came back, with the gift basket for the nursing unit in hand. He had outdone himself. It was filled with a multitude of little snacks, from healthy to just delicious, and several of my books.

Finally, we were ready! Despite COVID, everyone was giving hugs, with our masks on. True to my word, I walked out, using my walker pole. I was unsteady and needed to hold Ken's hand, but this was important to me. We continued saying goodbye as we headed for the elevator.

We barely held it together. We got out of the elevator and found a bench at a secluded spot down one of the hallways. And we both cried. The culmination of the stress, worry and endurance of the last few months flooded us and poured down our cheeks. These weren't sad tears; they were tears of survival. I had made it; we had made it. I was going home!

As our tears subsided, we headed for the car. It seemed like forever since I had been in our car. Everything felt fresh and new, invigorating. I sat in the front seat, admiring being a person, just a person, not a patient anymore. YAHOO! I was not a patient anymore. I still had challenges and some of them would be with me for the rest of my life, but I knew I could manage. I was one of the lucky ones, I was going home.

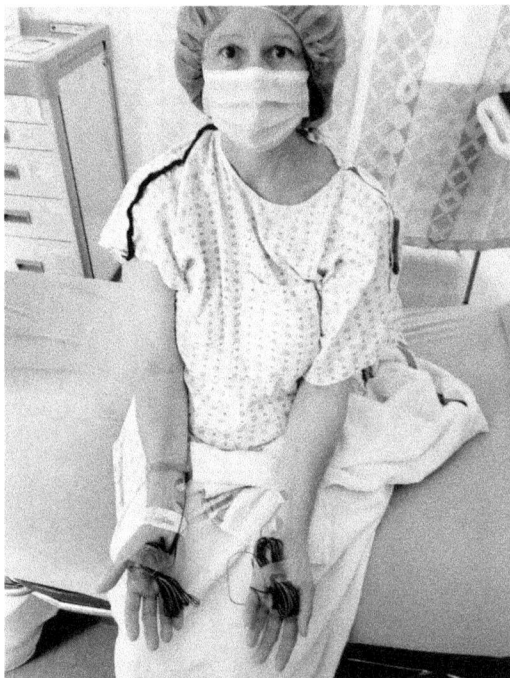

THE NEUROPHYSIOLOGIST JUST ATTACHED THE GEL ELECTRODES
IN PREPARATION FOR SURGERY. SHE'D ATTACH ABOUT 100 MORE
NEEDLE ELECTRODES ALL OVER MY BODY AFTER I WAS ASLEEP.

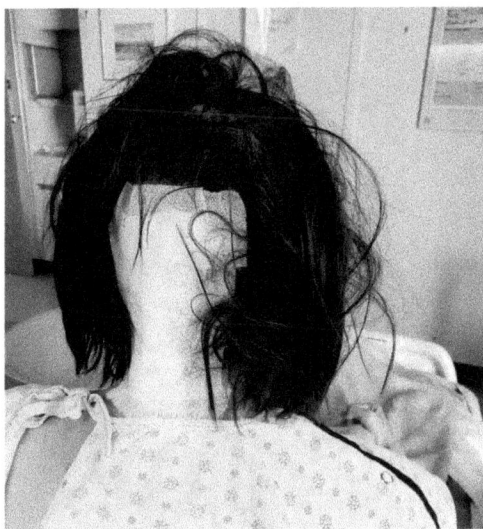

MY BANDAGED HEAD, STAPLED RIGHT INTO MY SCALP.

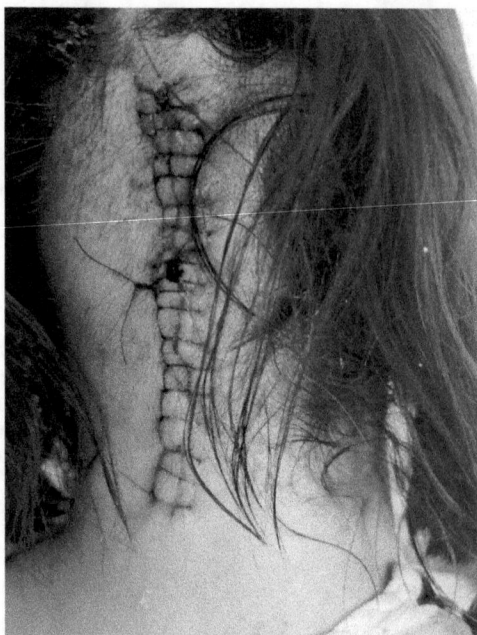

MY INCISION - FRANKENSTEIN HEAD!

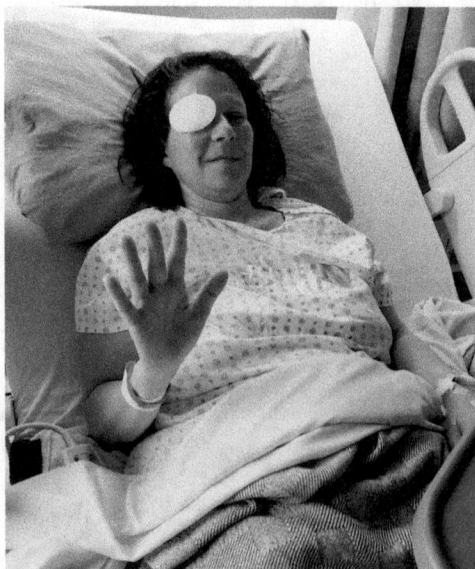

MY VISION WAS SO DISTORTED THEY COVERED ONE EYE SO I COULD SEE.

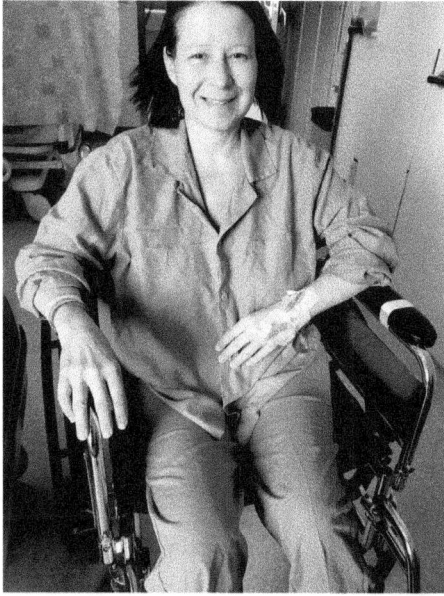

MY FIRST TIME OUT OF BED – AND INTO A WHEELCHAIR!

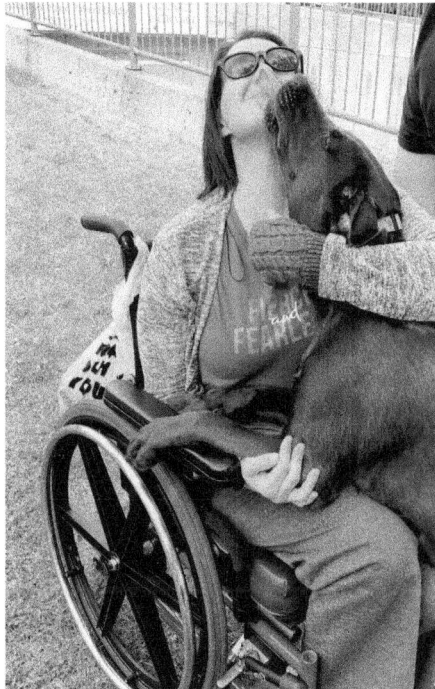

A SPECIAL VISITOR – ARTHUR!

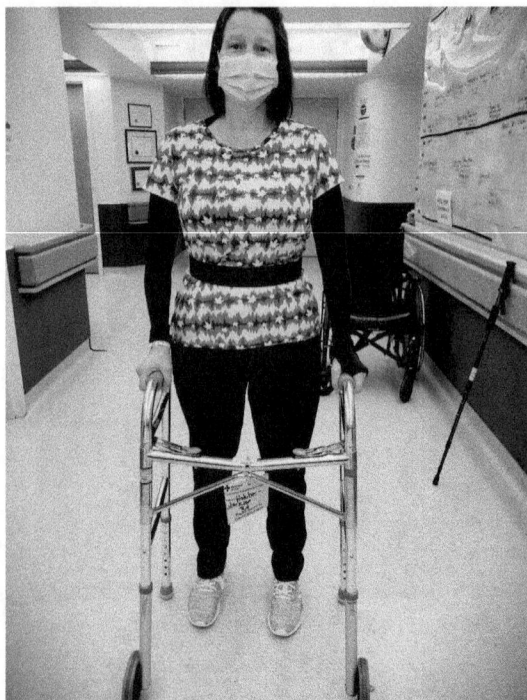

LEARNING HOW TO NAVIGATE A TWO-WHEELED WALKER.

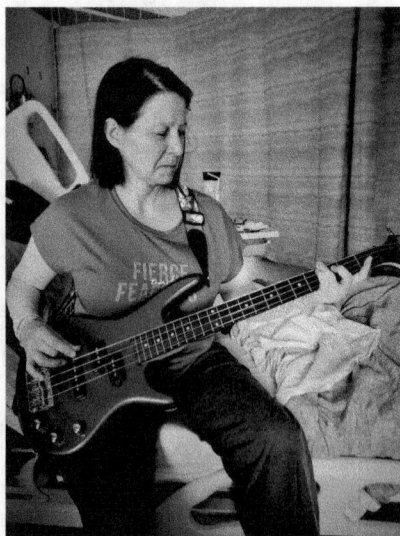

PRACTICING MY BASS IN THE HOSPITAL, COAXING
MY RIGHT HAND TO WORK AGAIN.

"It is not the strength of the body that counts, it is the strength of the spirit." J.R.R. Tolkien

CHAPTER 12

HOME

Being a passenger exacerbated my dizziness and vision. I went between wanting to see everything around me to needing to close my eyes to manage all the things going by. There was so much to see. There was a whole world outside the hospital, and I was a part of it again. As we got closer to home, Ken asked me what I wanted for supper. I had no idea. I hadn't needed to make any decision like that for quite a while. Now all the options of a grocery store faced me, all I had to do was choose.

A blank expanse greeted me when I thought about what I wanted to eat. Such a simple decision yet I couldn't think of anything. I felt mildly irritated that Ken hadn't just planned something, relieving me of this pressure. He was just trying to be kind, giving me a choice since for so long I had very little. I tried to think of something. It was so hard because my usually favourite, cheese was no longer an option. I couldn't eat cheese anymore!

Cheese was always my go to food, being a true cheese-aholic. Something changed since the surgery, and I just couldn't eat cheese anymore. Since that first time they gave me macaroni and cheese, shortly after my surgery and I couldn't eat it, I knew it was different. They offered cheese sandwiches for some lunches, and I found myself taking the cheese off. Me – a cheese addict! I wanted to eat cheese, I craved it, but when I tried to eat it, my body reacted telling me, in no uncertain terms: CHEESE IS WRONG!

Think about your most favourite food in the world, just imagine eating it right now. Maybe it's chocolate, or fresh bread, or loaded baked potatoes. Now imagine wanting to eat it but you just can't, your brain won't let you. It's crazy. All my flavour changes left me feeling undecided when it came to what to eat. What would it taste like? Would I like it? Did it matter? I think that's why I like my plain oatmeal so much. It's easy to eat and I don't have to worry about any flavours.

That's why the simple question of "What would you like for dinner?", caused me so much anxiety. I was probably one of the few who actually liked the hospital food. I suggested one of the meals I really enjoyed there, spicy black beans burgers, for supper. I knew we had some in the freezer before I left and thought they were probably still there. I was the only one who really liked them. The rest of the family would have beef burgers while I had my vegetarian ones.

Spicy black bean burgers it was. Ken made a quick stop to get buns and then we were home. Home! It had been so long since I had been home. It felt like everything had changed yet it was all still the same. The flowers had grown a lot, cascading down the barrels on either side of our driveway. The tree's leaves were fully grown, abundant in their foliage rather than still filling out. We pulled in and Ken helped me into the house. Emily was there to greet me as well as Arthur.

WELCOME HOME

My grand-doggy. He had come twice to visit me in the hospital and finally I was back. I was surprised how careful he was with me. His exuberance was usually warp nine, but now he was very gentle, almost cautious with me, not jumping, or bouncing around. He bowed his head and leaned on my legs, quietly whining for me to pet him. I felt myself getting emotional again. I was so happy to be home. Ken helped me to my spot on the couch. Emily and I chatted, Arthur laying between us, while Ken got supper ready.

The weather was still beautiful, the dry heat of end of summer prevailing. After a delicious supper, not served at 4:30, Ken asked if I was up to going into the backyard. YES! I could do what I wanted, I didn't have to wait for a nurse to help me, I didn't need to ensure I was back in my room by a certain time. I could have any type of snack at any time if I wanted. I didn't have to say goodbye to Ken tonight.

With some help I made it out into the backyard. It was beautiful. Ken did a great job, with his injured arm and his time spent with me at the hospital, planting flowers and gardening. We even had some tomatoes and hot peppers growing. The sun was still out, the grass was mostly green, and there were lots of birds flying about and singing. This was home. I relaxed into my chair and just took it in. Being able to smell the green growth, not surrounded by concrete and traffic was extraordinary. I love living in a small, rural town. I don't think I'll ever be a big city person.

Arthur was getting used to me being home and brought me his ball. We discovered another deficit I would need to work on. I tried to throw his ball. It went all wonky, hit a fence post and came right back at Ken. Every time I tried to throw the ball it was anybody's guess as to where it would go. We all laughed, it was funny and something Arthur would ensure I got lots of practice with.

Soon it was bedtime. My own bed. My own room, ahhhh. It was a delight. It's surprising how much we take for granted, every day. I was appreciating anew, every action, every element of our house. What I used to feel was ordinary and common I now realized how extremely lucky I was to have all this richness in my life. From our lovely home to a stocked fridge, to our backyard, to a family who loved me, I felt like the wealthiest person in the world. I don't think all this will ever become common to me again and I will always appreciate how much we have.

With our bedroom window open, feeling the fresh air, and listening to the frogs' croak, I fell asleep, holding hands with Ken.

LIFE BACK HOME

With the birds chirping outside, I woke up. I had slept so well. It was dark, cool, quiet. All the things I missed dearly while in the hospital. I was in my own bed, not a plastic mattress that always overheated me. Again, I am just complaining while still being so grateful for everything the hospital gave me.

Lying in bed, everything so familiar, my time at the hospital seemed like a blip yet it had dragged on forever. It's like climbing to the top of a very steep mountain, takes forever but in the end, it is so worth it. Every step you feel a burning in your legs, your feet are hot, your lungs, raggedly trying to draw in as much air as possible, never getting quite enough. You put your head down, concentrating on keeping your feet moving forward. Every time you look up, the top looks no closer, looming above, mocking you, so close yet so far. And then, the trees open up, and there it is, the top!

You are standing on top of a mountain. The sore legs, burning lungs, and sweat dripping down are all forgotten. Not only the view but the feeling of accomplishment, the pride you have in your body, you can't believe what it could do. The time, the hard work, the tenacity is worth it. The hours climbing up are forgotten in the satisfaction you experience in knowing you did it.

This is how I felt, leaving the hospital, being home again. There were times I wanted to quit. There were times I just wanted to go home. Not from the therapy but the challenges of being a patient and from being away from my home and family. Now that I'm home it seems like it was such a short time. I'm so glad I stuck it out, didn't give in to my own insecurities. I'm glad I kept at it until I could take in the view at the top of the mountain. It was worth it.

GETTING USED TO BEING BACK HOME

Ken heard me stirring and woke up as well. We stayed in bed, just appreciating being together. Soon, he helped me downstairs and made me a cup of tea. Then he helped me and we sat outside, it was a beautiful day. I missed this so much. Feeling the sun, hearing the birds, breathing the fresh air. I didn't have to ask three different staff, three times for something, I'm not hearing bells dinging, I can have breakfast whenever I want, I can have what I want, and I don't have to listen to the staff announcing my personal well-being. I'm probably exaggerating but sometimes it felt like organized mayhem. It was calm, quiet, and Ken knew exactly how I liked my tea.

Even good things take time to adjust to; a new job, a new baby, a new house, and there is often some work attached to it. Me being home was an adjustment for all of us. Ken didn't have to drive to see me anymore, but he was more worried when he had to leave for work as there was no one looking out for me. At the hospital I was safe, nursing staff were always there. The adjustments were minor though and soon the old conventions were settling back into place.

Every moment back home held special meaning for me. I was seeing everything through a new lens, one made of appreciation and marvel to be back in my familiar world. While still reveling in my gratitude, Kevin and Alix came for a visit. The last time Kevin saw me I was in a wheelchair with a huge incision on the back of my shaved head. My incision had healed, my hair grown enough to almost cover it and I could walk with my walker.

It's remarkable how much your world can change over the course of a season. But change is illusory. How much had really changed? For me it felt like everything was different but here I was, back in my home, enjoying my family, my garden, my home. What's the old saying, as much as everything changes it stays the same. I guess that's how I was feeling.

Soon my sister Cami arrived as well. We had a day with almost everyone home. It was a cool and rainy day, but the kitchen was filled with warmth and love. I was loving it. Too soon, Kevin and Alix had to leave. The school season was about to start so they needed to get ready for another year of teaching. I was glad Cami was still here.

We reconnected in a way that was missing over telephone calls and Facetime. Luckily, she made it just before COVID-19 numbers really started increasing. My sister Lydia would end up delaying her trip to see me because of unprecedented COVID-19 cases in the next few weeks.

One day I asked Cami if she could cut my hair. There was barely any hair in the back, where they had shaved it, but the front was much longer. I wanted it all to match it a little more. The day was sunny and warm, so we decided to do it outside, to lessen the mess. Arthur, only a year old, was full of silly antics, wondering what we were doing. Halfway through the haircut he grabbed one of the towels.

We let him have it as Cami was trying to concentrate on cutting my hair. Suddenly we heard, rrrrriiippp! If we weren't going to play, he was going to invent his own game, and ripping the towel seemed like a lot of fun. It certainly got our attention. We both broke out laughing and after a little chase and some treats Cami got the towel back. Sacrificing the towel was worth the laughs and the new haircut.

With the walker Ken had gotten from the Medi-lend we went for a short walk in the neighbourhood. We'd been living in our neighbourhood for eighteen years. We had incredible neighbours. A few came out to ask how I was doing. A few were driving by and stopped their cars to offer well wishes and welcome me back home. I felt so cared for.

The short walk and chatting wore me out and soon we were back home, appreciating some quiet time. Cami took over most of the cooking and we developed an easy, convalescing routine. She had brought fresh sage from her garden back home and made a delicious butter sage chicken dish one night. Cami understood on a deeper level what I had been through and was able to offer the support and help I really needed. It gave Ken a break too, knowing I was in good hands.

JAMMING

Several times, we all jammed together. Cami is a guitar player and singer, all self-taught. A few years earlier, while she and her husband were visiting, our band had a gig, and she was able to join us on stage and play along to Sweet Home Alabama. It was a very special experience. Now, with my right hand still improving, we were able to play some music in our jam space.

The practice I did while in the hospital really made a difference and I was able to play along to our songs. Cami and Ken took turns singing and I concentrated on playing the right notes. Wearing my earplugs to reduce the noise, I was able to play most of the notes and mostly in the right places. My hearing was still off but I find since my strokes and now brain surgery I hear music differently anyway.

When learning a song or practicing an old one, I don't really understand what I'm playing until I "see" the music. I've mentioned this before, and even wrote one of my newsletters about it. I can't stand a lot of extraneous noise but when I'm playing my bass in our loud band, I don't hear it anymore. I'm seeing what I'm playing. The notes are building structures in my mind. When the structures are built, I can play the notes. Luckily, in music many of the structures repeat, divided into verses and choruses. There's an added bonus, once construction is completed, I have it memorized. I just have to locate the right building for the right song.

Holding a pick is challenging but for most of our songs I just use my fingers. There are still times my fingers, hand and brain don't connect but fortunately, most of the riffs I play have solid foundations. I really missed playing music with others while in the hospital. It was reenergizing playing with Ken and Cami. Cami introduced us to a few new songs. We also played some old favourites including Ken's, "I Can See Clearly Now" by Johnny Nash. While playing it, Cami said the lyrics were made just for me and my journey through brain surgery.

The lyrics allegorically denoted being able to see a bright future because you had survived the worst of times. The rainbow after the thunderstorm had appeared, washing away the clouds and the pain, leaving sunny skies filled with hope.

Yes, those lyrics seemed written just for me. The obstacle was that malformation in my brain. It was now gone, and I could look forward to a rainbow, living life without the sword hanging over my head. Cami and I both had tears running down our cheeks. I saw Ken's eyes get watery too. I knew there were still some obstacles in my path but with the surgery behind me I was looking forward to blue skies.

As with life, time seemed to stretch on and then suddenly it was over. It was time for Cami to go back home. I was sad to see her go. Not for the first time and certainly not the last, I wished we all lived closer together. It seemed for so much of my life I lived isolated from my family. I had so wanted a close-knit family, but life had different plans.

Ever since we moved to Alberta, when I was just a child, I've felt a little displaced. I never wanted to leave Ontario. I had my grandparents, aunts and uncles, and cousins close by. I was the one who really didn't want to move here at all. It's crazy, my parents and sisters have all moved back to Ontario and I'm the only one left in Alberta. It is my home now and I've finally figured out, home is not a place, it's a feeling. I just wish we were all a little closer.

POST-OP APPOINTMENT

My eldest sister, Lydia was planning to come in a few weeks, so I had that to look forward to. Again, due to COVID-19, it had been a long time since we had seen each other. A few days before she was due to arrive, I had my post-operation appointment with my neurosurgeon. I was looking forward to it and letting him know how thankful I was for all he did for me.

Driving, or I should clarify, being a passenger in a car, was challenging. I couldn't drive. The stroke doctor at the Glenrose Hospital had informed Alberta Transportation of my stroke and surgery and had my driver's license taken away. It is protocol. Ken told me he had received a letter at home, notifying me I had to immediately go to registries and hand over my license. Ken was irked by this as it seemed insensitive since I was still in the hospital.

I'm glad he didn't tell me about it until later. I yearned for the independence that comes with the privilege of having a driver's license. I knew I couldn't manage driving though, as much as I missed it. Often, I had to close my eyes to combat all the visual input racing by when you're in a car. My double vision, nystagmus and dizziness merged together to create a feeling of being on a topsy, turvy rollercoaster instead of a highway.

At the hospital we passed through the COVID-19 security and made our way to his office. I was using my walker. I felt quite proud that I was able to walk there. Last time he saw me, I couldn't walk, at all. I could barely feed myself and needed help with every aspect of daily living.

After a short wait, he came into the examination room. We were all still wearing masks, but I could tell he was smiling. He asked a few basic questions about how I was feeling and how I was improving. I answered honestly and gave him updates from my time at the Glenrose Hospital. He seemed pleased and called my recovery "remarkable".

The doctor gave us an update on the surgery. He said he wasn't sure if he got all of the malformation. He told me that twice the neurophysiologist had to tell him to stop. Once because I had had two minor seizures and the second time due to the surgery affecting my heart rate. All that information runs through the brainstem, including respiration and heart rhythm. I wondered, just to myself, if all those bruises on my chest were from more that just the sternal rub to try and rouse me.

He recalled that there were a few tense moments when I wouldn't wake although he was confident it would be okay. To be sure, he took me for the emergency CT scan, himself. He even used the word miraculous with my recovery. Again, I realized anew how I didn't appreciate the seriousness of it all. Although I was doing very well, he cautioned that if he missed removing even one cell of the malformation it could grow back.

I took that to heart, but I knew the malformation was slow growing, at least I hoped so. The risk was monumentally reduced, and I could live with that, so much better than living with the sword over my head. I told him I was surprised about the titanium plate in my head. He casually informed me, no I didn't have a single titanium plate, I had four; each with two screws. WHAT! That was crazy, it seemed like such a small area. He brought up images of the CT scan to try and show us one. Unfortunately, since titanium is non-ferrous, it doesn't show well on the scans, but we were able to see one of the four fairly well.

In the area of brain surgeries, Ken asked if this type was a less common one. The neurosurgeon said that maybe one or two brain stem surgeries were performed a year in Alberta. I was again, speechless. I asked if there were any images from the surgery itself. It would be really interesting to see my own brain. He said a video was taken of the surgery that they used with the Chinese. The Chinese? I figured they must have a training agreement between our hospital and theirs.

The neurosurgeon went on to say he wanted me to have another MRI in a few months and then another appointment. If there were no changes the time between MRI's would increase but it was probably something that would be monitored for the rest of my life. That was okay, I was thankful for a life that needed monitoring. He also said I needed at least six months of a very quiet, calm lifestyle to ensure my brain healed. He also said a surgery like this required a full two years of recovery and a lifetime of adjustment to my newest normal. Again, I was okay with it and even expected it.

To ensure I would have the best recovery possible he said he would refer me to a Neuro-Ophthalmologist, to help with my vision challenges, probably the place I was supposed to go to from the Glenrose Hospital. Before we left, we gave him a thank you card although it seemed so small for the colossal gift, he had given me. We included several copies of our Glia Girl book on stroke. He seemed really pleased with the book and said he would like to share it with his colleagues in pediatric neurology. I was beyond pleased.

We left the appointment on a high note. I was so excited to be leaving the hospital, with Ken. Too many times I had to say goodbye to Ken from a hospital bed. No more, I was going home with him. I had told him this several times throughout the whole excursion; "I'm going home with you!" Once we were back in the car, I mentioned how interesting it was that they were using the video of my surgery with the Chinese. Ken looked and me, "Huh? What do you mean, the Chinese?"

I recalled our conversation with the neurosurgeon. Ken burst out laughing. After several moments his laughter subsided enough for him to tell me, "No, it wasn't for the Chinese it was for trainees!" Oh my gosh! I started laughing as well. I guess my hearing was still recovering. And it highlighted the importance of having a second set of ears at medical appointments. I was so glad I had not shared this with anyone else. Maybe that's how rumours get started.

RECOVERY AT HOME

I knew I still had a long road of healing and recovery ahead of me, but it was a road I was familiar with, and I knew I could do it. I had the tenacity and I had also learned patience, mostly. I still missed my old life. I always will. The only thing constant in life is that it will change. If it wasn't this, it might have been something else that changed. We had a good friend, we even did a podcast with him, about life change. He was an elite Ukrainian Dancer. A hip injury forced him to stop dancing and he was in continual pain. Life can steal parts of our identity, but it is also a good teacher that our identity shouldn't be too tied to the things we do, like our career or being a professional dancer. It is more ubiquitous than that. It's what's inside, our morals, values, the choices we make, our attitude that make us who we are. Every day, I am looking inside myself and trying to be a person I can be proud of.

The next little while we all worked on adjusting to my newest normal. Soon my other sister, Lydia, was coming for a visit. It would be great to see her again. It had been quite a while although with phone and Zoom calls the distance was well mitigated. Lydia ensured to send me a positive quote every day while I was in the hospital. It was very uplifting. I am blessed with such amazing, supportive sisters.

Then COVID-19 again changed our plans. Cases in Alberta were steadily increasing, causing unprecedented numbers. The hospitals were overwhelmed, and Intensive Care Units were filled beyond capacity. Even my neurosurgeon's office had closed half of their appointment rooms to use as emergency ICU rooms. The "Open for Summer" plan certainly backfired and the healthcare staff were continuing to pay the price. Sadly, but understandably, Lydia made the decision not to come out west from Ontario. We talked and it was the best and safest thing to do. She didn't want to expose herself through her travels and then share it with us. I didn't want her to get sick through her efforts to visit and support me. We would continue with phone calls and Zoom calls, just like the rest of the world.

As much as I wanted her to come, I couldn't bear the thought of her getting sick because of making the trip out west. Life is messy, full of unforeseen challenges and blunders. We had no choice with the increased COVID-19 cases, but we did have a choice in our response. We remained positive, knowing the visit would happen, just at a later time, when the risks were less.

My parents had postponed their visit until Christmas, hoping COVID-19 would be better managed by that time, but who really knew. Plans are made to be changed and the multitude of examples life has shown us only accentuated that truth.

I was taking it as easy as possible but my old, type A, busy personality was always lurking just beneath the surface. I would get frustrated at the things I couldn't do. Ken's shoulder was not functional, and we were still waiting for an appointment with an orthopedic specialist. Thanks, COVID-19. He tried but he couldn't keep up with everything that needed to be done. Sometimes it was easier for me at the hospital. I wasn't constantly reminded of the things I couldn't do; the schedule was set and there were no expectations of me beyond recovery. I'm not saying I want to go back, no way, EVER. Life isn't meant to be easy.

Not that my life was too difficult, there weren't expectations for me to complete work at home either, but I felt it myself. Seeing all the things I wanted to get done and not being able to do them was a constant reminder of my loss of independence, loss of ability. I tried not to let it get me down, seeking to infuse the lessons of the last four years into my well-being.

Most of the time I was successful. Going on Twitter was a huge help. Reading about other people's journeys helped me to be more compassionate to myself. Recognizing some of the shared struggles I had many "AHA" moments. I found myself developing an online community and learning so much about other parts of the world.

While Twittering I would catch glimpses into other cultures and lifestyles. It's those moments I realized how limited my world experience was. There are so many other cultures that are completely different than my own. My employment held moments of enlightenment as it boasted a multicultural workforce. I always appreciated learning about other people's cultures. It was like a light going off or an epiphytal moment when I comprehended how vast our world was. It is all encompassing and captured my thoughts.

Every time I've had the privilege to read someone else's life experiences that are so unlike my own there are always threads that share a commonality that I can relate to, bringing me closer to the author. Most of those threads include the importance of family, of caring for others, of social justice, education and pursuit of always trying your hardest to be your best self while giving back to your community, even to the world. It was and is very inspiring and despite differences in culture, beliefs, religion we are all more alike than different.

On Twitter, I read about many other people's brain injury recovery journeys. They were so open, honest, raw, and courageous. It really helped me to be gentler with myself and all I have endured. One poignant comment on Twitter said this:

"My friend asked me, - why do you keep talking about brain injury? Because brain injury is about your personality, the mystery of life, family relationships, equality... it's about being alive!"

As I mentioned before, having a brain injury is a fundamental change to your core. Maybe that's why there are so many survivor stories about stroke.

At home, to manage both mine and Ken's needs we developed a casual routine. I would do my Twitter posts and reading, do my exercises, and help where I could. I was starting to be able to do more cooking. I love cooking and was more creative due to both the time I had and constantly trying out recipes where I could find some flavour. My taste was still very reduced and with my new dislike of cheese, cooking had to be creative.

One of my new favourites was hummus. I love spicy hummus and added more flavour in the form of hot pickled peppers. Yes, I still love hot pickled peppers. There is just something about them that is so appealing. I eat them almost daily, that and Frank's Hot sauce, and siracha, and cayenne pepper, and just about anything else with a spicy element.

With all my love of spices, surprisingly, I love oatmeal. Just plain oatmeal. I ate and still eat it almost every single morning for breakfast. Dizziness is my constant companion. It's usually worse in the mornings, and I often find myself a little nauseous. After about an hour or so after I wake up, I can eat my oatmeal and it always sits well with me. When I've tried to eat other foods too early, I feel just yucky. I'm a good brunch person, but only plain oatmeal if it's for breakfast.

Ken was appreciative that I was doing more of the cooking, although he often mentioned the spice level was a little too ambitious. I got in the habit of ensuring he or Emily tasted my meals while I was cooking to help with the spice level. Previously I had never been too much of a fan of Asian type food. Now, I love it. Many recipes are more flavourful and most importantly, there's no cheese. I was still trying to navigate eating without my usual go to.

Besides food and cooking we developed a routine for taking Arthur out. I was still navigating with my walker and slowly increasing my endurance. I couldn't take Arthur on my own. I felt bad. Before my latest stroke we were walking buddies, using either my pole or the running stroller. The new routine had him out for one walk a day. Often, Ken would load up my walker and we would go to the nearby Rodeo grounds.

The times we went no one else was there and it offered a huge space for Arthur to run and chase his ball. The grassy field was flat, and I could push my walker on it. We went almost daily. I saw my stamina slowly increase, from fifty meters to one hundred and so on. It felt so good to be out in the fresh air, walking and watching Arthur run about. Most walkers offer a seat for resting and mine was no exception. I could take a break whenever I needed it.

On some weekend mornings, we still had our favourite routine. We would go to Tim Horton's. I would get my beloved steeped tea and a plain old-fashioned donut. Ken would get his coffee and something else, whatever struck his fancy that day. We would also get one plain old-fashioned TimBit for Arthur. We'd park at the rodeo grounds, drink our beverages, and enjoy our treats.

I loved this routine, I loved getting out of the house, appreciating the quiet nature of the Rodeo grounds. I am grateful to live in a small rural community that offers something like this close to home. I am definitely more of the country mouse than the city mouse.

AUTUMN AND THANKSGIVING

Fall was warm and beautiful, as only a fall in Alberta can be. The geese were gathering in huge numbers, getting ready for the journey south. I love the changing seasons and as I drew in a breath of the autumn air, laced with the scent of fallen leaves, I was so grateful to witness another one.

Soon it was almost Thanksgiving, being in early October here in Canada. Usually, we went to our good friend, Lucy's family farm. We had been going there for many years, decades. We met when we both lived in the mountains in Grande Cache, raising our children together, making memories and building a firm foundation for an everlasting bond. After many years, coincidentally, both our families moved to Fort McMurray within two weeks of each other. Our friendship was etched in stone, from all the shared memories and the comfort of knowing we would always be there for each other.

Through our friendship, we were welcomed into her whole family. Her sister-in-law became the keyboard player in our band, with us since its inception. Life's convoluted paths hold many surprises and golden moments, demonstrating the unseen connections in many events that seem to have no relevance to each other at all.

Unfortunately, there would be no Thanksgiving celebration at the farm this year. The explosion in COVID-19 cases ensured everyone stayed within their own bubbles, yet again. Travel within Canada was still allowed though, and Kevin made the decision to come to spend the weekend with us. His wife, Alix, would go to her parents. Although I was worried about him travelling, it would be so nice to have him home again. He assured me they would both take extra precautions, wearing N95 masks on the plane and such, and they were both double vaccinated.

I probably should have asked him to stay home, to stay safe, but I was so looking forward to spending more time together, I welcomed his visit. Our last two visits were overshadowed by impending surgery or regaining life at home after my extended hospital stay. This time Arthur remembered Kevin and greeted him with lots of tail wagging, kisses and happy whining. Emily was between jobs and would be home for the weekend as well. It would be a wonderful weekend.

The best part, we were able to bring back an old favourite we used to do every year, once we had moved to Wetaskiwin. In our yard we had two beautiful apple trees. I loved having the fresh fruit and always ate lots of apples, made pies, apple crisps, canned apple sauce and froze apples to use during the winter. This year, since some of the new changes brought on by brain surgery, I couldn't eat enough of the fresh apples. They were delicious and no longer had the salty tang I had tasted since my first stroke.

Ken had helped with collecting apples, as much as he could with his injured shoulder. We were still waiting for an appointment with an orthopedic specialist. We always had more apples than we could use, especially this year since both Ken and I were limited in our apple picking. We were able to get enough to bring back an old favourite, apple baseball.

We would collect the fallen apples and go to a nearby field. One person would pitch the apple, and another would smash it with a baseball bat. We didn't run bases or anything, the goal was to break that apple into as many pieces as possible, sending bits of sticky apple flying everywhere. We all wore old clothes, knowing we'd be covered in juice and apples afterwards. It was great fun. Later, the deer would come and eat up all the apple chunks. I participated as well as I could and had fun with the revelry.

Over the weekend we had many special moments and lots of laughter. I tried not to dwell on the absence of my eldest daughter, having no response from an email I sent her. Emily was still in contact, and I was hopeful that may lead to more for the whole family.

We made our traditional Thanksgiving turkey dinner, complete with biscuits, gravy, stuffing, and pies for dessert. I still had a very limited sense of taste. I remembered a scene from one of the Harry Potter movies when the children were invited to a ghost party. They served food but most of it was overripe or rotten. I sometimes find the over-ripe food more appealing as I can ascertain some flavour. Rotten though? No. Or I should say, not if I can help it.

Once, I was finishing my tea and was surprised, and disgusted to find lumps in the bottom of my cup. I checked and sure enough the milk had gone bad, curdled. I couldn't taste it, so I didn't notice until I reached the end of my cup. I'm a lot more careful with my food now. If I'm unsure of something Ken or Emily checks it for me.

The Thanksgiving weekend went by way too quickly. Why is it that the good times always slip through our fingers like soft, dry sand and the unpleasant times seem to be made of sticky, gooey slime that you just can't get off your hands. Kevin was headed back home, and we resumed our usual schedule.

"What If? … Every day is filled with what ifs?" CHJ

CHAPTER 13

WHAT IF...

Finally, Ken had an appointment with an Orthopedic Specialist. It would be in November. I was due to have another MRI in November as well, and another appointment with the neurosurgeon. Then in December, I had my first appointment with the Neuro-ophthalmologist. It would be a busy month and then some, of appointments. Emily was busy looking for a job that would be something she could do long-term.

And then she surprised us. She wanted to move to Edmonton to be with her older sister. Where did this come from? Kaylyn still wasn't talking to us or answering emails, but Emily was going to move in with her? It happened so fast. We tried to ask her to slow down, but to no avail. She was moving.

There was nothing I could do. I had to let her go, good or bad. It was her choice. I used to be quite a micro-manager, or as my husband liked to say, a control freak. I am learning, through life lessons that offered no choice except for my response. I am learning to let the chips fall where they may. I only have control of my choice and I need to stop feeling like I can control what happens in my children's lives. I need to let go and let them be themselves.

But what if something bad happened? What if my wonderful baby girl stopped talking to me too? What if??? Every day is filled with "What Ifs". My imagination can conjure up a thousand "What Ifs" in a nanosecond. The scenarios of my "What If's' kept increasing in direness until I worked myself into a complete panic. I've always been a worrier, especially for those I love so deeply but since my brain injury my worry has increased in tandem with my "What Ifs."

Letting go of my worries and my need to control is a hard lesson, but I'm getting better. I had no control when Kaylyn left, and I had no control when I was in the hospital. I just had to trust that things would work out, one way or another. I always wanted to protect my children, never let them experience hardships and heartaches. Therein lies the problem. Life is heartache and hardship. That's where we build our strength, our character and learn life lessons.

This is where they would learn to become the best they could and live their best lives, in spite of me and all my mistakes. Being in the hospital and not able to manage my own household was a very good teacher for truly learning this important life lesson. It's been a difficult one. Life is fluid, life is change, life is learning to go with the flow while still choosing your own path.

I always wanted to be a mother. When we were kids, we used to play the boardgame "Life". I always wanted lots of little plastic pegs that represented children in the back of my car. I was amazed at the miracle of each of my children. I wanted to give them the best of everything. Having three children is expensive and I had to work. I felt guilty going to work, then I felt guilty when I enjoyed parts of my career. I was so conflicted, trying to manage both. I was so tired, often foregoing sleep to ensure everyone's needs were met.

My stroke ensured I slowed down. I had to retire from working but by this time my children were mostly grown. I could look back at all the years of trying to manage motherhood with working and see the road of the past filled with every mistake I made, and it broke my heart a little more. But life is full of mistakes, or as I like to say, heartache and hardship. I made the choice, again, to not let all my self-doubt and past mistakes ruin me. I tried to keep my face turned towards the sun and chose to keep going.

MY THOUGHTS ON MOTHERHOOD

Being alone with my thoughts can sometimes be a very dangerous place. They go down some pretty dark alleys where mayhem is lurking in every dark alcove just waiting for me to truly let my guard down. Sometimes it feels easier to stay wrapped in a cocoon of despair because you don't have to try or hope or care. You won't be disappointed. But we only get one life, and I was so fortunate to have had several second chances at mine. I had a responsibility to make it my best life.

I'm trying to do the right thing, that's what is really hard and often really hurts. Being fully alive and living your best life isn't about being happy though, it's about feeling everything, learning from it, adding another layer to your character. It's about making choices and standing by them, even when it seems the world is falling apart around you. Like Westley, from the "Princess Bride" says, "Life is pain, Highness. Anyone who says different is selling something." I owe it to myself and all the people who have woven my cloak of care to make the most out of my gift of life. I don't know what will come next, but I am trying to trust myself that I will handle it and make the best choices.

I need to live now, not wait. I feel like I have been waiting for so long. First it was waiting to see if I could return to work, then waiting for a better recovery, then the next appointment, then this, than that. The list went on and on, even waiting for when the next bleed would come. I'm tired of waiting. Life is here and now, this very minute. In the lessons of life, I feel like I'm a very slow learner.

In one of my virtual newsletters, I talked about comparing decisions in life to the experiment with Schrödinger's cat. Schrödinger's cat was a thought experiment that illustrated the paradox of quantum physics. An experiment to prove that two realities could exist at once. Schrödinger left his cat in a box with poison and until he opened the box, he didn't know if the cat was alive and well or had eaten the poison and died. The cat existed in both states until Schrödinger opened the box.

I had recently read about an idea similar to Schrödinger's thought experiment that all time exists simultaneously; past, present and future.

It coexists in a fashion we are not able to comprehend. It exists like this to encompass every single event or outcome that could possibly occur. What we do or choose in the past affects our present and helps determine our future. The path is already laid out before us, our entire life, but how it unfolds in actuality is dependent upon us, our actions or inactions.

It's up to us how we make our choices, how we see or listen to signs set before us, which ones we decide to follow. I find this line of thinking very comforting. It means I was always meant to have this abnormality in my brain, and it was always going to challenge me at some point in my life.

The differences are beheld in my choices. Maybe I could have pushed myself to return to work after my first stroke and perhaps literally worked myself to death. Many times, I could have succumbed to the depression that links arms with life altering events, locking myself into the brume of my own mind, ruining what was left of my family.

I could have chosen not to have the surgery, living in fear of another bleed. Bad things happen. The important part is how we choose to react and handle these injurious life events. Knowing that perhaps every possible outcome has been predetermined gives us the control we have nowhere else in our life. It's up to us which reality we live in. There is no luck, no superstition, no horoscope that is going to determine my future. It's all up to me.

It's engrossing and beyond my ability to understand. It exists in the fringes of my capacity to comprehend but there is an inkling that this is correct. Maybe one day I will gain some understanding. Ancient people didn't understand what the Northern Lights were and took them to be portents of future events. Maybe in considering this concept we are the ancient people.

These intriguing thoughts swirled around my mind. Living in a state of always waiting and wondering what might happen was a perverse kind of thought experiment that I needed to stop performing. I needed to choose to live for today, every day. What choices we make determine which future we will live but we won't know what our future will really be until we make that choice and work towards it. What happens to the choices we didn't make; do they still exist somewhere else? We just don't know until we open the box to see if the cat is alive or dead! Perhaps some things aren't meant to be understood. I have learned that making the choice to be grateful to wake up and welcome a new day is a very good start to finding the future I feel I'm meant to be in.

LYDIA'S VISIT

Some days the choice to face the sun was a lot easier than others, but good things were on the horizon. Before all the appointments and while managing my youngest baby leaving home, Lydia was finally able to come for a visit. COVID-19 cases had stabilized a little and she felt she could manage the risks associated with flying. Her visit was like a breath of fresh air. She opened the windows of our privations and brought in a fresh breeze that carried much needed love and laughter.

We talked, made memories and also made my famous rum-soaked fruit cake that took a full three days. After it was baked it then needed to be fed with rum, every five days, for another six weeks. We played games, she went for walks with me and Arthur, and gave Ken a break from worrying about me when he had to leave the house. It was a wonderful time. I was open about our struggles and pleased for an understanding ear. I was again reminded that Ken and I weren't alone, we had people who loved us and wanted to help. I was filled with gratitude renewed.

The week flew by, like that soft, slippery sand in an hourglass and all too soon, we were saying goodbye. The memories would last forever, as would our sisterhood and friendship. She left with her own fruitcake and memories. As she departed all our appointments began.

APPOINTMENTS

The first appointment of many was my MRI. I had had lots. This would be my ninth. I still didn't like them, but I was prepared. At least I didn't need to have a contrast MRI. Contrast is when they inject a dye intravenously into your arm during the MRI to enhance the quality of the images. It also allows the radiologist to read the images more accurately. A doctor prescribes the contrast to be used during an MRI. I was glad not to have it as it doubles the length of time the MRI takes.

The next week we went to Ken's Orthopedic appointment. It was as we thought. He needed surgery, ASAP, to repair the three muscles that had detached from his rotator cuff. They wanted him to have an MRI and then he would see an Orthopedic surgeon. They were fast-tracking his appointments, realizing how long he had been waiting. One doctor mentioned he should have had treatment sooner. He smiled apologetically, he knew the reasons behind the delays, all too well. At least now Ken would get the care he needed to repair and heal his shoulder.

An interesting turn of events happened during that appointment, and several others I attended for Ken. When the doctors saw me using a walker, they inquired about it. When I told them about my craniotomy, in my brain stem, the response reminded me of the seriousness of the surgery. The doctors were quite interested, and we spent several minutes talking about me and my surgery. I wasn't trying to steal the limelight from Ken's appointment, it just happened.

Then we were off to my neurosurgeon visit. I don't know what we were expecting but we were a little disappointed. I think I was hoping for a definitive "all clear" no more malformation, no more risk. Unfortunately, that was not to be. It was healing nicely but there was still residual blood and blood products in the area obscuring the images in my most recent MRI. He was not able to see or say with certainty if he had removed the entire malformation.

With memories of him telling us it could grow back if he even missed one cell, we left his office. He was pleased with my recovery, still calling it remarkable, but also coated it with caution. I would continue to improve for the rest of my life, but I also needed to accept my new normal. We felt a little heavy-hearted. We knew that my risk was greatly reduced, and this is what we really needed to embrace. Appreciate each and every day with conviction!

RECOVERY GOES ON

Not long after I was watching a show about extreme athletes. I found it fascinating. Before my strokes I always wanted to complete an Iron Man competition. I had even made a deal with myself that if I did finish one, I would get the Iron Man tattoo, on my ankle. I would never complete one now and I had made peace with it. I was grateful I could walk but I still love watching shows about these elite athletes.

In this particular episode the extreme athlete was talking about what it took to complete the death-defying physical challenges he was doing. He kept comparing the intensity to digging into the deepest part of your brain stem to find the tenacity to complete them. He kept mentioning the brain stem, specifically. He also said that pursuing and surviving his extreme feats were transforming physically but mostly mentally. I found this very interesting. I wasn't doing anything even remotely close to what he was, but I survived several injuries and surgery right in my brain stem. Maybe this was the life changing part of my journey. I'm no extreme athlete but I am a survivor and coming this far has been transformative and transcendent.

Prior to strokes I was an avid runner, completing several full and half marathons and even two Death Races. Maybe this is part of my penchant for documentaries on extreme athletes. I was never a top finisher or anything close, but I did enjoy running in events, the camaraderie, the support and yes, the post-race food. I loved training too. I feel that my training has been very helpful in all my stroke recoveries.

I was familiar with the hard work it took to increase your distance and time when running. You had to take it slow and build on prior runs or risk injuring yourself. It took time and discipline and repetition. With longer runs, it took mental fortitude, to keep going when all your muscles were screaming at you to quit. I applied the same strategies to my stroke recovery. I took it slow, built on prior training sessions and saw improvements. It's a much different type of progress, but it's progress. I've also learned to listen to my body. I can't push myself like I used to, or my legs and arm will just stop working, I get even dizzier and more nauseous.

I've come a long way even though I measure my distance in meters rather than kilometers.

Soon it was Ken's turn for an MRI. He had never had one and was a little nervous, especially since he is a big guy. He's not claustrophobic but the idea of being squished into a metal magnetic tube was cause for consternation. I gave him the goods on what to expect from all my MRI's. The worst was he would need to drive there and back since I still didn't have my driver's license.

The MRI was as expected, and Ken survived. He found the experience quite uncomfortable but managed alright. The healthcare staff were very kind and helpful. He was glad it was over and was looking forward to the surgeon appointment. He was also a little more understanding and sympathetic to all my MRI's. Walking in someone else's shoes is the best teacher. We received word that the appointment would be in January, just after Christmas. More waiting, poor Ken.

MY EYES

One more appointment and then it would be almost Christmas. I was looking forward to seeing the neuro-ophthalmologist, really hoping there was something he could do so I could work towards getting my driver's license back. As much as I knew I wasn't ready, I really missed driving. I hoped for the chance to at least try. Experience was on my side to earn back my license, having done so much driving with my daily commute. Mine had been revoked since my brain surgery, standard protocol for anyone who has a neurological event.

That it was standard procedure didn't make it any easier. My license had been revoked after my first stroke as well but at that time I was able to return to driving with just a doctor' note. This time, the stroke doctor had informed me, due to my condition, I needed to attend the driver retraining program at the Glenrose Hospital. It was an interesting program, designed to help people return safely to driving. I had seen some of the equipment they used when the therapist used virtual computer programming as part of my therapy. For the driver retraining they had a mock car with screens all around to simulate being a driver. It was a good way to start, ensuring no accidents or injuries would transpire before getting behind the wheel of a real vehicle.

Once they deemed the person efficient and safe in the simulated car, they had a real car and a small training course in the underground parking lot. I couldn't wait to get the okay to try and get my driver's license back. Me, who used to commute over 700 kilometers a week just to get to work. Me, who also had my mobile crane operator's license, and had no problem driving a standard.

When you think about how much a stroke takes, it is something else. But, as always, you can't focus on the negative. I was grateful to have Ken, ever so supportive, as my chauffeur. He told me, anytime, just ask, and he would take me wherever. I joked that I would get him the typical chauffeur hat, with the name "Chives" embroidered on it. I don't know why but that seems like a good chauffeur name. The real problem, and it's my problem alone, is having to ask. I hate having to ask. Not having a driver's license, when you're used to driving, takes away a huge part of your independence. I try to be realistic though, I couldn't even go shopping by myself.

There is so much I can do; driving is such a small part of my life, but I was looking forward to the appointment with the Neuro-ophthalmologist. I knew there was no magic formula to improve my eyes and dizziness, but I was hopeful that he could offer something for a little improvement.

We arrived at the hospital where the Eye Institute of Alberta was. It was a large, very active clinic. There were all sorts of ophthalmologist specialists, not just neurology. They also received all the emergency eye referrals for central and northern Alberta as well as northern British Columbia, Saskatchewan, and the Northwest Territories. They had several waiting areas depending on who you were seeing and for what. They even did a variety of day eye surgeries, including repairs and cataracts. It was huge and a far cry from the small clinic with the optometrist I visited with Kelly's Taxi when I was in the Glenrose Hospital.

After a short wait an eye technologist came for me. Ken was able to join me. She was very friendly and efficient. She performed the standard eye tests including testing for colour recognition. It was thorough and afterwards she led Ken and me into the main exam room. Then a neuro-ophthalmologist resident came in. The clinic worked with the University of Alberta and had a strong commitment to training medical doctors to become eye specialists. She was bright and bubbly and the future of specialized eye care. While conducting a multitude of tests she told us about the accolades of this eye institute.

She claimed it was the best one in Canada and considered herself very fortunate to be finishing her residency there. She also talked about how much she respected the neuro-ophthalmologist I would soon be seeing, sharing what a wealth of knowledge and experience he was. Her testing took about 45 minutes, and I was starting to feel the effects of all the eye strain. Then the main doctor came in.

I don't know what I had built up in my mind, but he was nothing like what I expected. He looked to be in his late sixties, with a head full of silver hair. He had a quiet, kind demeanor and was extremely polite. He spoke softly and explained things as he did them. He gave off a vibe akin to Mr. Rogers. I instantly trusted him. He reviewed the residents' notes and then did his own testing, including freezing my eyes, putting dye in them, and using some kind of microscopic assistance.

I didn't understand all the tests, but I sure felt it, especially the tracking tests. My eyes jerked and jumped all over the place. He assigned my condition with a plethora of very long words like, nystagmus, oscillopsia, binocular diplopia, vertigo (that one I understood) and some others. Then we got to the meat and potatoes of the appointment. Was there anything he could offer that could help and would I be able to attend the driver's retraining program?

With his kind and gentle demeanor, he said there were special lenses he could prescribe that would help, called prisms. Prisms help mostly with double vision (diplopia) by aligning the images so only one is seen. Prisms work by the way they change the direction in which light is reflected. Prisms trick the eyes into believing an object is in a different location in order to improve eye alignment. He tried some with me and they did help. He clucked his tongue and softly said I should consider waiting before moving toward prisms.

It had only been six months since my surgery and the doctor didn't want to start using prisms as it might affect the natural healing and re-programming of my brain. As much as I wanted to drive again, I knew that I wasn't ready. I accepted what he told us and appreciated it when he wanted me to come back in six months for another checkup. With my trust in this kind, gentle specialist, I knew he was looking out for me and my eyes and wanted the best recovery I could have. It was still frustrating though. I had perfect 20/20 vision, but I couldn't "see" properly!

"Pain is inevitable. Suffering is optional. Everyone has sadness but at some point, sadness becomes a choice." Anon.

CHAPTER 14

LIFE IS A ROLLER COASTER

Our last appointment before Christmas was complete. Although I was disappointed it felt right to wait longer before I attempted retraining. We had to go to Motor Vehicle Registries to turn in my driver's license. We were finally abiding by the very stern letter sent while I was still in the hospital demanding I hand in my license within ten days. Ken was affronted by the tone of the letter and reasoned that since I wasn't able to return it myself, he'd just ignore it. We forgot about it but realized I probably needed current photo identification other than my passport, so we went and returned my license and I applied for the government issued ID.

It was a little heartbreaking, giving up my license but in the whole big picture of what was going on in my life, it was a pretty small crack. I wasn't yet giving up hope on one day returning to driving either. I was learning, again, to be patient.

To fill the time and my thoughts, I started doing some baking, as I could, for Christmas. My heart really wasn't into it. Emily was still with Kaylyn, and it seemed her mental health was causing her more challenges. Kaylyn still wasn't talking to me, and the situation was just so inimical. I also had the feeling that my parents would cancel again. COVID-19 numbers had reduced slightly but the risk was high, and many people were still hospitalized. My intuition was correct. Two days before they were supposed to come, they made the difficult decision to spend Christmas at home. As much as I was disappointed, I understood. I wanted them to be safe and again, couldn't stand the thought of them getting sick trying to visit me.

Christmas was complicated. My family was fractured, the weather was cold, and we couldn't participate in any of the usual Christmas merriments due to COVID-19 protocols. Since the Christmas Eve when Kaylyn told us she had eloped, Christmases have been hard. Upon reflection, their elopement was such a trivial thing. Again, hindsight is twenty-twenty. It's like my vision, it's 20/20 yet I still can't see properly, just like you can't change the past.

EMILY BACK HOME

Not long after Christmas, on a cold minus thirty-five day, Emily moved back home. Things had gone extremely sour between Emily and Kaylyn and her wife. I'm still not sure of what all happened. It was an amorphous situation. I think Kaylyn's wife was transitioning into a man so perhaps I should say husband. I don't know enough about any part of it so I'm not sure. I welcome the opportunity to learn more about their own journey.

There has been a lot of media attention over people who are gay, lesbian, transgender or gender fluid, or something other than heterosexual. It often takes me by surprise when I hear on the news that people who are part of the LGBTQIA2S+ community are subjected to discrimination. I don't understand everything, but I am willing to learn and more importantly accept. What matters to me is that you are a good person; being kind, caring, not wanting to cause harm to others, that's what counts. How you express yourself or dress or who you love is your business. My good friend from the steel mill is engaged to a woman, and I love them both for exactly who they are.

By creating biases and singling out anyone who is different we're just increasing the divisive nature of humanity. By making it a big deal it becomes a big deal when it never should have been. Why can't we just accept each other. If someone has a need or a calling to express themselves in a way that is different than ours, why can't we just embrace it and celebrate our individual uniqueness. If we were all the same, what kind of world would it be.

People we have called geniuses throughout history, like Einstein, Darwin, and others, challenged our way of thinking by promoting what they believed. History called them ahead of their time, pioneers in learning. Sometimes they were called heretics, or even dangerous. Their genius and need to discover and be who they were was an innate part of them. Other scientists followed in their footsteps, no longer afraid to research taboo subjects. Perhaps this is the same for the changes we are seeing within the LGBTQIA2S+ community. People are becoming braver in sharing who they are meant to be.

When Kevin was in high school, he told me that music was more of a passion than soccer. He was on an elite competitive soccer team at the time. As talented as he was at soccer, music was and is a part of who he is. We have to embrace those parts of us, let them out so we can be who we were meant to.

For me, stroke unleashed my desire for writing. It was always there, even in grade school, but somehow stroke let it truly come out. When I get an idea or inspiration, I can write thousands of words without even stopping, the words falling out of my head and into the computer. If we don't let these integral parts of ourselves out, they may start expressing themselves in ways that are not healthy. Perhaps Kaylyn's wife, now husband, has embraced what is truly their identity. Unfortunately, I am guessing but hopefully one day we can have an open discussion about this.

I was happy to have Emily back home, but she needed more help than I could give her. Luckily, she was receiving some professional therapy and I prayed it would help her. We all went through another transition time. Learning how to live together, find strategies for mental health, live within the overshadowing world pandemic.

THE DARK MONTH

January was a dark month. My thoughts were imbued with dark feelings, and I was having bad dreams again. Nothing like my previous dreams. Since my brain surgery my dreams are not so vibrant or memorable. Mostly just bits of images. I had survived three strokes, brain surgery, a gang attack on our house, losing my career, losing my daughter, and so much more. I was and am a survivor. I would not, could not, let this take me down. I have a responsibility not to give up. I have been given another chance for a reason and I have to live my best life to give back to show my gratitude for my renewed opportunity. This is something I could not waste by wasting away.

Several years ago, Ken, Emily and I had a painting night, painting wooden plaques to hang in the backyard. We all put a favourite saying on our plaques and mine was "Ad Astra Per Aspera" a Latin phrase for "A rough road leads to the stars". As I recalled that night and what I had painted it gave me comfort. Maybe my convoluted path through life was leading me to the stars. It lent me some fortitude to keep going.

With that in mind, I did what I did best. I got busy. I was more active on Twitter, reading and posting inspirational passages, hoping the words would infuse me with the faith, courage, and optimism my world was lacking. What do they say, fake it till you make it. I was faking it, for sure. I had another Glia Girl Adventure in the works. Ken supported me so I engaged myself wholeheartedly with that, I started building my story and researched the topic, which was concussion.

After I was satisfied with the story, I wrote up descriptions for the proposed illustrations. I sent this off to our amazing illustrator. She was happy to provide us with her talent for our second book. I was grateful. Her illustrations breathed life into my words and brought the story to full colour. I was excited to see them.

I also started picking up more responsibility with my volunteer position with Covenant Health. They had given me the time I needed to recover until I felt ready to resume my role. Thankfully all the meetings were still virtual so I could take part from home. All added up, it was only about four hours a month but enough to fulfill my sense of purpose.

From my volunteer position on the board other opportunities blossomed within Covenant Health. I was able to provide a video for things like "What Matters to You" day and join in a "Lunch and Learn" explaining the important work our council did elevating patients to be valued members of their own healthcare team. I loved the work and the team I was a part of. Everyone was so kind and supportive. It helped give my life direction and fulfill my mission of giving back.

The seasons continued and soon the days weren't so dark and cold. Finally, COVID-19 had abated just enough that my parents felt safe to come and visit. It had been such a long time since we had seen each other face to face. We were all fully vaccinated, and my parents were very careful during the flight, wearing N95 masks the entire time.

MY PARENTS

It was so good to see them. I hugged them as hard as I could, trying to make up for lost time and missed hugs. We all had tears in our eyes that spoke words we could not say. It was a beautiful visit. We didn't even miss not being able to go out or socialize with others. We stayed nestled in our little bubble of COVID-19 safety and reconnected after such a long absence and all the mayhem that had ensued.

They had aged, or so my mom said, mentioning how old they looked. I didn't see any of that. When I looked at them, I saw the two people who had always been there for me my entire life. I saw the love, the support, the constant care. The other stuff, the grey hair, and other signs of aging, disappeared. They are the people who are always there for me, no matter what.

All too quickly, it was time for them to go back home. As much as I wanted them to stay, it was time and we had things happening. Finally, Ken would be getting the much needed surgery to repair his shoulder.

Eleven months after he had torn three of the four rotator cuff muscles right off the bone, he would be having the necessary surgery.

We met with the surgeon. He instilled a feeling of confidence and trust. He was open and honest, even telling us that since so much time had passed, he wasn't sure he would be able to make the repairs 100%. He did assure us that he would improve the movement Ken had with his arm and shoulder. Luckily, it would be day surgery.

Since I still wasn't driving, and Ken wouldn't be able to, we asked Emily for help. She had just started a new job, improving in her mental journey enough to get back to work. We were so happy for her and the strides she was making towards her own health. If she couldn't get time off, we had a plan B in place. Luckily it was no problem.

KEN'S SURGERY

After so much time the day finally arrived. We woke early and Ken drove to the hospital. With COVID-19 protocols in place, only I was allowed up to the pre-surgery area with him, and only long enough to see him settled. They didn't want any extra people around, potentially sharing germs. I left him there, with feelings of a role reversal since my surgery, less than a year ago. With the help of my walker, I went back to Emily who was waiting in the car.

We went for breakfast and found ways to pass the time while anxiously waiting for the call that the surgery was done. It took all day, but we were kept up to date, knowing that the delays were caused by Ken not yet having the surgery, not some other calamity.

There was such a backlog of these types of surgeries. They called it an elective but that didn't feel accurate. I guess elective surgery is because the surgery can be booked in advance, it's not a life-threatening emergency. It is life changing though. Ken was looking forward to being able to use his right arm again. It had been such a disadvantage for him over the past eleven months. If he could get even seventy percent increased mobility, the surgery would be worth it.

Finally, we got the call. Ken was in recovery, it had gone well, and we could pick him up. Emily drove to the patient pick up area. She would go in by herself. With my walker, I wouldn't be able to help Ken into the car. I waited anxiously. Soon they arrived. I tried to help as I could. Ken was wobbly and showing the effects of whatever medications they had used.

We got Ken settled and started for home. We were still in the city when Ken promptly got sick. Emily was in busy traffic, I was trying to get a bag for Ken, Ken was speaking nonsense words. Somehow, we managed, with minimal mess and maintaining our safety. The rest of the forty-five-minute drive home was uneventful.

Once home, the rest of the evening and that night were very quiet. Ken even slept well, the medication still wrapping him in a cloud of painless bliss. Then morning came.

The surgeon had warned that he was going to cause Ken a lot of pain. He wasn't wrong. Fortunately, he had prescribed some efficient pain medication. We made sure that Ken took it regularly, to keep the pain at bay. To manage the discomfort and the awkward positioning of his arm and shoulder, Ken ended up sleeping on our reclining couch for many nights after that first one. Ken used the technique Cami had taught us, visualization, to focus on having a functional arm instead of the discomfort of recovery.

Day by day, Ken's arm slowly healed. Two weeks later Ken was supposed to have a post-operation visit. Emily was unavailable. Our good neighbour, who had offered was only busy the day of the appointment. Our plan C backfired as well. Ken and I didn't know what to do. We came up with a solution that probably wasn't our best idea, but it worked.

Ken would try to drive himself. I hooked up his seatbelt and changed gears for him. We took the country roads, avoiding high traffic areas. We made it safely. I tried to do as much as possible to support Ken, even managing to take my walker out of the car, with a little help from Ken's good arm. I was still using the small one Ken had borrowed for me from the Medi-Lend before I got out of the hospital.

The appointment was quick but not rushed. The surgeon was happy with Ken's progress and even gave Ken some beginning exercises. He mentioned how he wasn't sure if he would be able to fix it at all, just because so much time had passed. The muscles that were ripped off Ken's rotator cuff had atrophied and receded down from his shoulder towards his elbow. The surgeon was worried they wouldn't be strong enough to be pulled back up and reattached to the rotator cuff.

Thankfully they were. I had four metal plates in my head and now Ken had three little posts on his rotator cuff where the surgeon reattached the muscles. What a pair we were. The surgeon was very pleased with Ken's progress. He said Ken would probably have close to full range of motion once he was fully healed. He also said healing and physiotherapy to regain strength and movement would probably take a full year. We were getting lots of life lessons for patience.

KEN'S RECOVERY

Ken wasn't bedridden but was restricted in what he could do. The weather was still chilly, with snow and ice on the ground, even though April was approaching. We weren't able to take Arthur out on his usual walks. Emily took him out when she could, but she was still getting used to her new job. I would take Arthur into the backyard, but the ice was such that I couldn't even throw the ball for him.

The walker we borrowed was not capable of navigating the icy and snowy sidewalks. The vibrations from the little hard wheels were more than my dizziness could bear and they constantly got stuck. These types of walkers were designed for flat, smooth trails; something paved or mall walking. I hadn't yet taken Arthur out by myself, but I knew he needed to expend his energy. My running stroller, that Ken had gotten for me before my last stroke, was still in the garage.

I pulled it out and decided to try taking Arthur for a walk on my own. Ken was concerned but necessity is the mother of invention, or so the saying goes. In my case it provided the push I needed to become a little more independent. Arthur was over a year and a half old now and just barely settling down. I practiced walking with him inside first, up and down our hallway. While holding onto the stroller, his leash in hand on the handle, I felt confident I could manage.

Ken was nervous and made sure I had my phone with me. I also had a pocketful of treats to ensure good behaviour from Arthur. I was excited and was surprised to be more than a little nervous too. Off we went. It was just a short walk but a revelation in my recovery. I could do this. One small step towards renewed independence. Both Arthur and I were very happy.

We started going every day, just for short distances. We're fortunate to live on the outskirts of our small town. Not far from our house are big fields and open areas. Often there was no one else around, especially when the weather was poor, as it often is at the end of winter so I could let Arthur off the leash so he could really run. It was great therapy for me, and Arthur could expunge his exuberant energy.

The running stroller was very good, enabling me to go places I couldn't with my walker, but it still bound me within confines of my own disabilities. Walkers offer a seat for when you need a rest, and rural central Alberta had many challenges on the trails and very few benches. My dream was to go off trail, maybe even return to hiking one day. The running stroller couldn't quite make it.

One day, trying to navigate an uncleared snowdrift, the front wheel fell off. As much as society has improved with access, winter comes with inherent challenges, exacerbated for someone with mobility issues. I had my phone and could have called Ken. Instead, I sat on the cold ground and figured it out. It was straightforward and soon I had the wheel back on. Pushing it on the bumpy ground had loosened some screws. Fortunately, they were right there, and I didn't have to search for them.

I returned home both happy that I fixed the stroller myself and frustrated that the wheel had come off in the first place. I wondered out loud why someone hadn't invented a walker for people who still wanted to be active and have adventures. There is a stereotype that if you need a walker, you only want to go on gentle walks, no more adventures. That's not true, I still want to go out and I'm sure many people with mobility issues feel the same way. With that came the realization that I hadn't even looked to see if something like that existed. It was time for a Google search.

NEW WALKER

I started researching and typed in, all terrain walkers, not having much hope. Then I found it! A link to a website that boasted all terrain walkers. "The Trionic Veloped – A Modern Alternative to a Rollator!" I clicked into it, a feeling creeping up my spine, telling me this was it. The more I read the more excited I became. The first sentence read – "If you lead an active lifestyle, the Veloped is your ideal choice of a wheeled walker." It went on to tout its ability to negotiate tough terrain, saying the three-wheel design was more off-road capable than any four wheeled walkers[3].

Could this really be true? A walker designed for people who still wanted adventures. A walker for exploring and taking the less travelled trail. It had a special extra wheel in front to climb curbs, roots and other obstacles and proclaimed it turned "gravel, grass, snow and off-road trails into pure pleasure instead of a bumpy and unpleasant venture." They even had a model specific for hunters to "overcome rugged hunting ground."

Two obstacles, that were not on the trail, stood out. The one company that had the foresight to offer people with mobility challenges all-terrain walkers was in Sweden. The second, being such a specialized device, they were cost prohibitive. I couldn't get the thought of this walker out of my mind though. I was always a very active, adventurous sort of person and I was sorely missing it. I didn't want to be constrained to smooth, even paths forever.

There is always a way. Ken discovered that the company had a distributor in Canada. He contacted them and found out the Veloped was, in fact, a medical mobility aid. He then contacted his insurance company and they said, if it was deemed medically necessary, they would cover a

---

3   Here is a link to find the All-terrain walkers.
     https://www.trionic.ca/en/veloped-%E2%80%94-the-alternative-to-a-rollator-i-18

portion of the cost. We went through the process of getting it authorized as a necessity and voilà, we ordered the Veloped.

Surprisingly, it only took three weeks to get here, all the way from Sweden. They didn't have the one I needed in stock in Canada. It was a breeze to set up. The designers thought of everything. It was so user friendly. In minutes we had put it together. I rolled it around our house. The special design had it climbing up the small step from our sunken living room. Now I could really explore the fields behind our house with Arthur.

It worked like a dream. It had a little backpack and storage area. It even had a waterproof cover for the storage area, truly capturing the vision of the designers. I could carry anything we might need. It had a comfortable seat so I could rest whenever I needed to. The brakes were strong and easy to use. The first time I used it, my friend was visiting, and we went out. With its' large, air-filled tires there was hardly a vibration from the bumpy ground into my hands and arms. I was even able to easily push it up a curb to access the path after crossing the road. It was amazing. I am so thankful for this company that had the vision to realize that needing a walker doesn't mean the end of outdoor adventures.

Arthur and I went walking every day. Arthur was getting used to the walker and walking right beside me. He knew I would let him off the leash when it was safe. Slowly my distance increased. I was thrilled to have a little taste of my independence back. There is always a way even if it's different from what you envision; if it works for you, it works. The new walker certainly worked for me, and I couldn't wait to try to it on some real trails.

Ken was continuing to improve. He had another visit with the surgeon scheduled and with the success of the last one we didn't even try to find someone else to drive. The surgeon was still pleased with Ken's progress and told him he could start with physiotherapy. Things were going in the right direction.

MY BRUSH WITH COVID

Things were going really well, and then I got COVID-19. A brief encounter with someone who didn't know they was infected was all it took. I self-isolated within the house, as best as I could, wearing a mask when I left my area. Five days later Ken came down with it. Emily did too and had to miss work. Luckily, maybe, Ken wasn't missing work as he was still off, recovering from surgery.

Ken and Emily had a fairly mild case. I got all the symptoms and then some. I felt awful. My limited sense of taste and smell was completely obliterated. My whole body was achy, and my dizziness exacerbated. It would be weeks before I felt better. Poor Arthur, again his walks took a back seat.

With seeing how contagious COVID-19 was (and is) and listening to the news about our fragile healthcare system being tested beyond its limits, and now experiencing the disease firsthand, I felt a new frustration at the Freedom Trucker Convoy that had happened just after Christmas but was still making headlines in the news. I was fully vaccinated and believe that if I hadn't been I would have been one of those people who ended up in the hospital, maybe even on a ventilator. The whole situation has been very divisive as well as concerning. It brought out a lot of strong emotions and continues to.

As I've said many times, life is messy, life is full of mistakes, life is full of taking chances. We see this everyday in the news. I witnessed it firsthand in my own life. I guess the best we can do is try to maintain our own personal circle of peace. Things were settling down at home and we were all finding our own rhythm, finding some peace again, with Emily back home and Ken's recovery after surgery (he was doing very well). I still tried to keep in touch with Kaylyn, writing her emails. After the dissolution of her and Emily's relationship Kaylyn answered once in a while. It progressed into scheduling a phone call. I was so excited and so nervous.

*"Be careful of your moods and feelings, for there is
an unbroken connection between your feelings and
your visible world." Neville Goddard.*

CHAPTER 15

KEEP GOING

When we finally talked, after so long, it wasn't anything like I expected. Initially I was just holding back tears at hearing her voice, so familiar, so beautiful, longing to just take her in my arms. I didn't want to scare her with the intensity of my emotions. I made two crucial mistakes. I was so worried about saying something that might offend her or scare her off I didn't tell her anything I was really feeling. Second, my heart was so broken I had to wrap it with a little protection. I was guarding it and so that also kept me from saying what I really wanted to, what I should have.

We had one more phone call and I tried harder. I still found it so difficult to be myself, to be her mother. So much had happened, I didn't even know where to begin. I told her I loved her, and we chatted about safe subjects, nothing delving too much into the personal. It was like I had cotton stuffed down my throat, the words were so hard to get out. I was stuck in this place between telling her how much I missed her and being afraid of her never calling me again if I said something wrong. Panic and anxiety took my words. Trying to find the right words while dealing with a brain injury made it even more difficult. I wanted to keep trying, hoping to start building the steps to a renewed relationship, but she stopped answering my emails again.

I remember reading the Eragon series of fantasy books. I loved them. They were all about magic and dragons, good versus evil. If you haven't read them, I don't want to ruin it but one spell the hero uses on the enemy is a spell of understanding. I just want Kaylyn, all my children, to understand, even though I've made mistakes, I always loved them and only wanted the best for them. They are so important to me. My brain has changed making all this chaos even harder to understand and process. I wish I had some magic spell to right all the wrongs.

I was a young mother, only in my twenties, but I felt so ready. All I wanted was to be a mother. During my pregnancy I was filled with love, excitement and a confidence that belied my age and experience. If I knew then what I know now, it would have been very different. The love wouldn't have changed but I would have the benefit of more life experience. Living life is how we gain that treasured experience. We can't go through life looking back and wondering what could have been. We have to be open to learning from our mistakes and moving on. That's how life works. To use a well known comparison, that's why the rear-view mirror is so small and the windshield is so large. We're meant to look forward, towards today, tomorrow and only glance behind us to ensure we remember the lessons learned.

Life is scary and precarious. My job as a mother was to protect my children. I did it too well. In protecting them I didn't give them enough chances to just figure things out for themselves, learn from their own life lessons. I can't try to think I know how they feel or think or dream. This has been the hardest lesson of all, letting go, letting the people I love be the people I love them for. Stroke has been quite a teacher.

With all the mayhem my new normal created there were times I isolated myself. I truly felt stroke, brain surgery, everything I had been through really brought on all these family challenges. I wasn't a good enough mother, I couldn't keep my career, I couldn't even keep my driver's license. In a warped way I felt I wasn't worthy of having and keeping friends. Why would anyone want to be around me? During some of my really low times I believed I was a failure.

MUSINGS

All these things wrapped up into an ugly parcel containing any self-esteem I had left. But having a child leave you is beyond comprehension. It shakes you to the core. If your own child doesn't seem to love you, are you worth loving? It takes all your confidence. I can't find the words to convey the depth of my grief, of my sorrow. I try not to talk about it much, it's easier that way. What can I say if I don't have any words and how can I explain it if I can't find any answers?

A few years back I read a book our friends, Lucy and Rob, had given me. It used to be Rob's mother's. It was a collection of personal stories from people who had survived the Great Depression. The stories were filled with hardships, tough choices, and incredible tenacity to survive unbelievable poverty. Some families had to make the hardest choices imaginable. They had to send their older children out to survive on their own so the younger ones would have a chance of living. The older children were sometimes only twelve or thirteen years old.

There are many examples of families torn apart by war and famine. I used to work with a lady who left all four of her children in her home country so she could find work to send money back to support them. It had been years since she had seen them, but she knew she was doing the best thing for them to have a chance for their future. There are so many stories of families whose circumstances have reduced or obliterated their contact and communication.

Maybe I am making too much of my own situation. We all have a choice and Kaylyn has made hers. I just have to find a way to deal with it. I read several books that address this exact issue, children withdrawing from their parents, their entire families. It is not as uncommon as I thought. I realized I was quite naïve in my world view, thinking children and parents would always be there for each other. One of the books described estrangement of any kind as the worst punishment out there. In fact, some cultures use banishment as a reprimand.

It is so hard to manage my sorrow and I feel I can't openly share my grief. I'm grieving the loss of my daughter while she still lives. My greatest fear is something severe really happening to Kaylyn and I won't even know. I'll hear it through the grapevine months later. The smallest tidbits I hear from social media or the few friends we know mutually give me such a great relief. Occasionally, Kaylyn will have brief contact with my sisters. As much as it hurts, I am grateful to hear she is at least alive!

As I've said before, reading posts from other stroke survivors really helps. Many are still coping with the life changes decades after. I feel there is a direct link to the changes in my family and my stroke. The saying goes that correlation is not causation, but I feel these two are correlated and the latter was the cause. I need to learn patience with my recovery, so I need to with my family as well. Maybe I just need to toughen up? I don't know. I let my thoughts ramble in relation to who I am and my new normal.

I've endured so much and I'm so grateful for my second and third chances. I'm not going to let life's adversities change who I am. My passion to help others and give back won't change. I will not become a hardened bitter shell. I am a survivor and although stroke has affected parts of me, that one fundamental core of my being that wants to help others hasn't. No, just the opposite, it fulfills my soul to help others. I strongly believe it is more than just who I am, it is my responsibility, one that I bear happily. I have a debt to pay, for all the gifts I have been given, for all my chances to live again. The old adage, you receive more when you give rings true.

My life has taken such a different path than I ever could have imagined pre-stroke. Things I'm doing now I never thought possible. Things I can't do anymore also seemed impossible. A friend made a poignant comment, "Our health is great until it's not." The original quote is from Thomas Fuller, "Health is not valued until sickness comes." I think that is what my friend meant. I certainly fell into that category. I took good health for granted. Although the path has been diverted, I believe it is the path I was always meant to be on. My life has completely changed but I feel it is a good life.

But am I a good person? I'm trying to use my time wisely, trying to help others. Who decides what is good, who are the judges of goodness in our crazy world. If you watch television or any type of social media, the definition of good is as capricious as the snowflakes falling during a winter storm. From the many books and online posts I have read about other people's journeys, I know the only one who needs to feel goodness in me - is me. As with my stroke recovery, it is a journey I will be on for a long time, probably for the rest of my life.

One lesson life is teaching me is to talk less, it's been a hard one to learn. I love talking and I love languages. In my early life we had a family joke when my grandmother, who didn't speak English very well, called me a motor-mouth for talking so much. I used to feel that any problem could be solved if we just used the right words. Life has taught me, yes, words are important but there is so much more. Sometimes saying nothing is the best course of action. Sometimes doing nothing as well. I'm still learning my lesson of letting go and thinking I can control things. I wanted to control things with my words. I have learned and say a lot less now.

I used to believe in magic in the world. Not a witchy magic filled with spells, hexes, or curses but a magic of words. Words that could paint a picture, weave a tale, offer solace, even hope. Jesus used words to teach, offer hope and insight into ways to live for a better future. His many parables imparted a multitude of valuable life lessons. The wisdom within them is still shared today.

Sometimes the despair of all I have lost makes me feel my words no longer contain any magic. I speak the words, trying to repair the damage of living but the magic I used to feel my words could deliver has evaporated, having no effect, offering nothing to those that hear them. Words have the power to uplift and heal but as with any power, words also have the ability to hurt, destroy relationships, break hearts.

With all these life lessons, maybe I better understand the evil characters in fairy tales, how they were created. Maybe they had too many black words used against or towards them and they had to harden their hearts to survive, to keep them from breaking anymore. I'm not living in a fairy tale, and I am responsible for my own happy ending. I'm learning and despite all I've lost I am trying to hold my head up, look towards the light and rebuild my self-confidence. Where is the young woman who had to learn how to curtsy to accept an award from Prince Michael of Kent![4]

Some days I'm strong, I can manage the monumental number of unexpected changes in my life. I know it will be okay and I have hope for the future. It's like President Snow in the Hunger Games, "The only thing more powerful than fear is hope!" Hope is a very dangerous thing. There are some days when hope seems to overpower fear and sadness. I love those days, everything seems easier. Other days, the hope is too thin, like sea foam being dissipated by continuous waves, not able to hold onto anything at the whim of the strong ocean current.

I'M OKAY

I've created a façade of being okay, that I really haven't changed that much, that I still see the sky as blue. It's a thin veneer. Building and maintaining the veneer is a continuous process, it is constantly cracking and I'm constantly trying to repair it. Ken can see through it. He knows about the veneer and the many cracks. He tries hard to offer balms to keep it whole, keep me whole, to give me time to repair the cracks once more and keep going.

Evenings can be difficult. If I had a hard day, whether doing too much or the emotional tolls of life, by evening I see everything as a disaster. Not only are my physical symptoms exacerbated, but my ability to process my thoughts also evaporates. It feels like my world is ending. There is no hope left. I've now learned when I get this way the best thing to do is just go to bed. Life will feel right again in the morning, and I can keep going.

I owe it to myself and the many people who have contributed to my cloak of care. I'll keep saying it, I'm a survivor. It's funny how much things change, though. A favourite quote Kevin and I like to share states, "The more you learn the more you realize how much you don't know."

---

[4]   In 2003 I received an award from Prince Michael of Kent for my work with the Life Saving Society.

I am a firm believer in that quote. I've learned so much since my first stroke, but I am still just a babe in the woods. There are so many lessons to learn and often relearn. I'll read a passage from a book that offers sage advice, and it will be like an epiphany. It makes so much sense.

Life is one big classroom; life is one continuous learning adventure. A lesson I've learned anew is what really matters to me. In my first memoir I shared my bucket list at the time. We all have some kind of bucket list, things we want to do or accomplish before we die. There was even a movie about it, the characters embarking on all sorts of daring adventures.

My bucket list included several things, including awesome life adventures. I look back at it and realize how much it represented how I was still feeling at the time. I was still in the initial phase of accepting my new normal - "Our health is great until it's not!"

I feel or maybe just believe that I have accomplished two of my bucket list items. One was to write something others would want to read. I think some people have appreciated reading my first memoir. I also feel that my Brainy superhero in my first Glia Girl Adventure Book has been successful, so far. We'll see.

My second item on my original bucket list also included my desire to make a difference in the world, even a small one. I don't know if I'm making a difference in the world at large but I do know I'm trying to help others. I am so grateful for my work on the Patient, Resident and Family Advisory Council with Covenant Health. It allows me to use my experiences to try and help others. I didn't think I would have this much "patient" experience though! Covenant Health also offers many other avenues for helping and I participate as I can.

I have a new bucket list now. It has only one item. I want to have my family back together. I want us to be able to have a supper where we exude kindness and respect. I want us to reminisce about good memories, leave all the hurtful ones behind. A bucket list of my other items is superfluous to me now. Many of the items listed in my first memoir really demonstrated how naïve I was and how little I had accepted my new normal. I still thought I'd be getting my old self back. Don't get me wrong, all the things on that previous list I would love to do, and some I might, in a modified fashion. But they are no longer bucket list worthy. I really only have that one item.

After my first stroke I had written notes for my funeral. I'm not thinking about funerals anymore. It's too macabre and I'm trying to focus on life. Funerals are not for the deceased anyway. Their worries are over. They are onto a new adventure in the afterlife. Funerals are for the ones left behind, the ones trying to manage the loss of a loved one. A funeral allows people to share their grief and find support and comfort. The one who has passed is now at peace, their troubles, pain, and struggles, are over. But perhaps funerals are necessary for the ones missing the deceased. I don't know.

J.R.R. Tolkien had an inspiring way of describing death and dying. In his third Lord of the Rings Book, the character Gandalf imparts these wise words, "Death is just another path, one we all must take." I have always been a big fan of The Lord of the Rings and J.R.R. Tolkien books in general. I find one passage or perhaps concept, that Tolkien describes in a few of his books, very comforting. Even after the ring is destroyed and Middle Earth is again filled with peace, the wounds Frodo, one of the main characters, has endured throughout the story are not healing. Time does not always repair all wounds.

To find peace in his life and a chance to rest and replenish, Frodo is offered the chance to heal in Valinor. Valinor is a mythical place that could be described as what people might think of as Heaven.

"...and it was blessed, for the Deathless dwelt there, and there naught faded nor withered, neither was there any stain upon flower or leaf in that land, nor any corruption or sickness in anything that lived; for the very stones and waters were hallowed." J.R.R. Tolkien, The Silmarillion.

As Frodo journeyed there, he again felt goodness enter his heart. I believe Tolkien was very wise in describing a journey to and through death, using his fantasy world to bring a clarity to this enigmatic thesis; death is not the end. Those who loved Frodo were greatly saddened but they were able to say goodbye before he left. I feel it was a very ingenious and spiritual way to describe our beliefs for the afterlife and managing the sorrow of losing a loved one.

COVID-19 has changed funerals. What would I want? Mmmmmmh. Although Frodo's sendoff sounds beautiful, it's not possible in our reality. Maybe I want something like in one of the Celtic songs we sing in our Band, "Paddy Murphy". It's a funeral full of shenanigans and drinking, more of a party than anything else. That would be great for people to refer to my funeral as the best party they ever attended.

I'm no longer afraid of death, I feel like I've been given several chances so every day I wake up, especially since brain surgery (I AM ALIVE) is a bonus. I'm not afraid to die. Like Tolkien, I really believe death is just the start of another journey, a place to finally achieve peace, heal, and who knows what opportunities and adventures may be awaiting me. I believe there is a grand design to the world, how could there not be? When I look at the incredible relationships around me within the natural world, there must have been some engineer planning it out.

In his book, "Natural Theology" Rev. William Paley of Carlisle made an argument that stated, "There cannot be design without a designer... The marks of design are too strong to be got over. Design must have a designer... That person is GOD."

One of his associates, Charles Darwin, explicitly tried to go against this train of thought but like many things in our world, maybe they can co-exist. Perhaps the designer provided a blueprint then life and necessity refined it; a continuous fine-tuning, happening even as I write this. Some parts of our humanness have barely changed over a millennium but other parts, such as how we live, how we interact with each other and the world around us have changed vastly. No longer are we hunters and gatherers. Science has explained much but not everything, hence the grand design. What happens after death remains a mystery, something beyond our capability to understand.

The thought of a grand design is a comforting one. There is some sort of plan within our crazy world. Even though the thought of death doesn't scare me, I'd really like to live long enough to see my family back together again. There's a song that really resonates with me, and on days when the sadness tries to overtake me, I recall these words, "There's a peace I've come to know …. No more sorrow, no more pain." I can hold on because I know my next adventure will bring with it peace for my heart.

Who knows if I'll ever see my bucket list item come to fruition, but I'll keep hoping, trying. Something I've learned, throughout my whole rollercoaster ride, death or near death really teaches you to live. That's another quote that really resonates with me, "You only live once. WRONG! You only die once; you live every day." As bad as things have been, I'll never give up. I'm living every day, grateful. And I want to keep living, finding opportunities to repay my renewed chance at life.

NEW SINGER

Another way I'm able to give back is through our music. I am so grateful I can still play my bass. While I was still in the hospital, not hearing properly and my hand not working, I practiced my bass. I may never be the bass player I was, but I can play well enough. The band hasn't kicked me out. I don't think they ever would. We are like family. We are lucky with our band family. Ken's shoulder had also healed enough for him to return to playing like he used to.

We had a new singer join our band. She has fit in so well and is sharing her talent with us and the people we are so fortunate to play for. COVID-19 finally receded enough that we could try our new band out in public. We were lucky enough to play several gigs. Ken is our band manager and has a gift for finding us gigs. Our one band, The Cod Tongues, plays mostly Celtic music. It is a novel niche that people really seem to enjoy. It is fun music that gets your toes tapping. I feel blessed every time we play for others, sharing our music.

We have a special bond created through playing together. We are a team, and the camaraderie is paramount. We succeed or fail together. There is no finger pointing or blaming. We are just like the slogan used initially for COVID-19, "We're all in this together." Playing music together really develops your ability to listen. There are so many cues throughout a song to ensure you play the right notes or sing the right words. If you're not listening to each other, you'll miss your cue and play out of time or incorrectly. It's a good life lesson that we're all trying to apply elsewhere; the value of listening to each other.

Being in a band is work too. Not just practicing the songs but set-up and take down. The music comes with a lot of equipment. I'm not able to help with the physical parts anymore. Luckily, I can help with organizing our songs and writing down any changes we make to ensure the music reflects what we play. Another life lesson, there is always a way and even if I can't do the physical parts of moving equipment and such, I can still help and be useful.

I appreciate being in the band in many ways. Besides the joy of playing music together, it helps keep me busy. When I'm playing, I'm not thinking about all the other things going on in my life. It is a balm for the many wounds my heart bears.

Sometimes all these thoughts, all these memories just get to be too much. I wish I had something like Harry Potter's Headmaster, Dumbledore had, called a pensieve. It's a magical device to relieve oneself of the burden of holding onto all the memories. In the book, Dumbledor uses the pensieve to store and review past memories when and if needed.

"I use the pensieve. One simply siphons the excess thoughts from one's mind, pours them into the basin, and examines them at one's leisure." Dumbledore in "Harry Potter and the Goblet of Fire".

I don't want to lose any memories. My memories are all my life experiences that have helped shape me into the person I am today. Who would I be without them? Sometimes my brain just feels too full, though. Pensieve's only exist in books, but perhaps writing for me is a little like Dumbledore's pensieve. Once I put thoughts down on paper or a computer screen, I try to leave them there. It is very cathartic for me.

That's the secret; finding what works for you. No matter how many self-help books you read, therapists you talk to, or remedies you try, nothing works until you do; until you are ready to move on, to make a change, take that first baby step towards the life you want. Often the help is there, just waiting for you to be ready to find and accept it.

It's amazing all the lessons to be learned from the people we interact with. People who smile, say a kind word, go about their daily routines and we have no idea what's really going on. Never judge a book by its cover, one of my favourite sayings, even more so as I'm going through my own journey. We don't know who is living with what, the pain they are experiencing, the black scars that life has painted on their hearts. I think everyone has a story, everyone lives with some pain, has some scars. Maybe that's the secret, making the choice to just keep trying. Affixing a smile, just trying to survive, hoping to catch those moments when the pain abates, just a tiny bit. A pain that is so constant that any amount of reprieve is monumental.

KEEP GOING

People who choose to keep going, to find the best in life even when it has shown them the worst encourage me to keep going. A family friend, who is also a priest, was a guest for one of our podcasts, "Faith and Healing". He shared a sage analogy. He said, to be able to accept help and move on we must have our car in drive, not park. If we keep our car in park, we won't be able to go anywhere. Kevin and I also share another quote that reflects this advice for life, "Hard work takes you to where good luck can find you."

Kevin works very hard and often finds good luck, the kind of luck that seems easy to others because they haven't seen the hours of work to get there. Kevin's hours of practice and extra work have brought him good things. Often when we see the work of true masters, they make it seem so easy. The hours upon hours of hard work, all the trials and tribulations they endured to achieve their mastery are shrouded by their virtuosities. When we see a true master at work, we applaud and celebrate their genius. Sometimes the opposite occurs, some people are quick to judge, so easy the masters make it seem, even if the critics themselves have no such skill to display.

Kevin is achieving mastery and I couldn't be prouder of him. All the turmoil within our family has affected Kevin too but he continues to have a positive attitude and very insightful thoughts on life. Since my first stroke, rarely does a day go by without him calling me. Only exceptional circumstances prevent a call and then we still text each other. There exists a confidence in our relationship that transcends words. He knows I will always be there for him, despite the mistakes I have made, just as I know he will never abandon me, even as he grows and lives his own life fully. I have learned so much from my son, the teacher became student when I'm with him.

Life has provided me with many teachers. There is so much to learn. The saying, "When the student is ready the teacher will appear" often rings true. I think sometimes the teacher comes many times but often we do not recognize these teachers of life until we are ready. When one of my teachers imparts their wisdom and I begin learning the lesson, sometimes it almost feels like a long-forgotten memory resurfacing, perhaps I'm recalling past teachers who tried to teach me. Other times it is like the proverbial light bulb going off. Some of the lessons are hard but I am grateful for every lesson and every teacher.

Another one of my teachers came shortly after my first stroke. I wrote about it in my original memoir. Back then I was not used to the slower pace that stroke had forced upon me. It was new and I started noticing things I previously had not had time for. From my spot on the couch, I watched some birds build a nest on the hedge outside of our family room. Those birds became my teachers. Here's an excerpt from *7 Jars of Hot Pickled Peppers* describing what I learned as I often needed reminders when life tried to pull me in too many directions.

"The couple (birds) started building a nest on the far side of the window giving me a great view of all their work. I could see them coming and going with various sticks, twigs, and bits of string in their beaks. I could see the little engineers constructing a sturdy home for their future children.

It was amazing to see how these first few twigs woven in the branches of the hedges started to take on the conical shape of a snug nest, effectively hidden from the larger birds. And they were accomplishing it with only their beaks, feet, and each other. I marveled at their tenacity and resourcefulness, and it gave me encouragement. I had so much more at my disposal to be successful and the birds provided a timely lesson. Building their nest was the foundation of their existence and it would take an extreme situation before they would deviate from their goal. I needed to focus on what truly mattered and give up my juggling. I found comfort in watching these busy birds and gained some inspiration for my own life."

This is a lesson I learn and relearn; focus on what really matters. There is so much extraneous noise trying to pull a person in a thousand directions. When I feel overwhelmed, I think back to those birds and focus on what really matters. I look at one thing, one twig. I can't start something else unless I have built a firm foundation of what I need and decide on the direction I want to go.

QUILTING

Learning to quilt was another lesson for focusing on one thing. My neighbour very patiently introduced me to the art of quilting. Quilting is very much focusing on one thing while having a plan for the future. You can't sew the whole quilt at once. You have to make one square at a time. It was the start of a great life lesson for me. At work we always talked about looking at the big picture. Sometimes the big picture is overwhelming. That's the trick, the lesson; focusing on one tree while not losing sight of the fact that there is a forest.

Quilting was such a good teacher for the lesson. I could focus on one square or row at a time. As I completed each one, I could put it aside until I finished the next one and was ready to start putting the quilt together. Even then it was a methodical process. One quadrant, then another. It emphasized the importance of taking big jobs that appear overwhelming and breaking them into small manageable chunks. It reflects another favourite quote of mine; "don't look at the whole staircase, just focus on the first step."

I found the process of quilting and the life lesson it presented so inspirational I asked my quilting instructor if she would do a podcast with Ken and I about it. She agreed. It was all about the benefits of hobbies but also about the process of breaking things into small steps. Kevin calls it scaffolding, building one skill on top of another. We called the podcast, "You Can't Eat an Elephant."

The quilting instructor was very nervous. On the first try, her nerves got the better of her. To be honest we probably rushed her into it. We smartened up for the second time. We knew my instructor and her husband outside of quilting class. We invited the two of them for dinner, including lots of wine. The wisdom just rolled off her tongue and we had an incredible podcast. As a funny aside, Ken and her husband sat in the back doing the recording and enjoyed some more wine. Everyone was smiling by the end.

She shared lots of insight. One pithy piece she imparted was that sometimes goals need to be readjusted. If a goal seems unattainable, don't give up, change it to suit your abilities and timelines so you can be successful. It fit in perfectly with the theme of not being able to eat an elephant. She shared other secrets of her life learning. Another favourite of mine is her telling me the value of sometimes pretending to be a little deaf. Sometimes people say things they don't mean or perhaps try to get a rise out of you. Pretending not to hear them is the best recourse and lets everyone go on with their day with no hard feelings.

We can just watch the daily news to see a plethora of examples from people saying inflammatory things to spark a response. Sometimes we should all be a little deaf. Like the old saying goes, "if you wrestle with a pig, you'll both get dirty, but the pig likes it." The message to me is, don't wrestle. It's so hard and sometimes it seems as if the whole world is going mad. Maybe that's contingent on what influences we're subjected to.

WHAT WE SEE

How we see depends on how we look. Perhaps it's our life experiences that determine how we look. We look with so much more than our eyes. As a child I looked at the world with wonder and beauty. Now, sometimes I see a world filled with pain and heartache and suspicion of ulterior motives. Daily I consciously try to make the choices to rediscover wonder, magic and beauty in our world. I'm living proof miracles still do happen. And I'm trying really hard not to wrestle any pigs and sometimes I need to be a little deaf.

It's challenging and now and then the roadmap of navigating relationships, recovery and living with a brain injury seems circuitous at best. Occasionally I feel like I'm on the doorstep of understanding, but I can't quite walk through. My thoughts drive me wild as I feel the answers are right there, just on the other side but I can't step across the threshold to turn them from the nebulous swirls just out of reach to comfortable knowledge within my injured brain. Sometimes I feel if I could figure out how to get through that door, even put one foot on the edge, I would be infused with the wisdom I feel I'm lacking.

At the heart of these thoughts, I think of how much I survived. Maybe without the twists and turns in my roller coaster ride of life I wouldn't be where I'm at in terms of understanding what's really important. I'd still be more type A, over-working, competitive, perfectionist, and yes, sometimes even a little judgey. I wouldn't wish my journey on anyone else, but I feel I have grown so much and perhaps I am a little wiser. I am so grateful for each and every day, even the hard ones. I'm trying to spread kindness and help others as much as I'm able. It's just so hard not being able to help my own family.

Whenever profound sadness threatens to overwhelm me, I go back to the basics of what I am grateful for and what brings me joy. Something as simple as being able to make my own cup of tea and drink it. I remember when I was in the hospital and couldn't do that.

I keep trying to figure out how to sand away the negativity, like in my dream and the evil figurine that I thought I could fix. There is no magic solution, but it might be that easy. Instead of sanding away the evil in your life you just need to make a decision, a choice, to find and concentrate on the good.

It's hard to choose sometimes. It's easier to stay in those low places. You don't have to try or hope or care. But that's our superpower, that's my superpower. That's where I have control and should use it with every ounce of my strength. I have to choose who I want to be in each and every moment.

With all the challenges life keeps throwing my way I need to dig deep into that well of strength to keep going. It's getting pretty deep, and the ground is getting harder but as long as I am alive, I will keep digging and finding the strength I need to keep going. That's the door I need to find the courage to walk through.

I have had bad days, and they are tough. I usually just retreat into myself without sharing when things are rough. As I've mentioned before, Ken can usually tell and encourages me to slow down, take a break, knowing I am a little fragile during those times. I've been through a lot and still carry some risk. The neurosurgeon is still not 100% certain he removed the entire malformation. I'm still under his care. I'm still having regular MRI's. I need to respect my body and take care of myself during those times.

Most people don't realize how hard I am trying to appear normal. I often need to avert my eyes to control my dizziness and diplopia. Sometimes my sensory sensations on my left side are so bad I can't stand it. Sometimes my left leg doesn't work, sometimes my right hand doesn't work. Sometimes I can taste a little, other times, nothing at all. Even though my speech is vastly improved, it still takes effort to find the right words, control my shaky right hand, or not to stumble. I don't want to constantly go on about managing my new normal, but I do need to be a little kinder to myself and not expect to be perfect and not show my true challenges.

I've worked so hard to regain what I've lost, several times now. Often no one sees my practice exercises. Sometimes even Ken would ask when the last time I practiced my rehab exercises was. I would tell him today, and he would be surprised! I'm improving and my goal is to keep improving. I think we are all doing some form of that. We all want to be the best version of ourselves that we can. But don't mistake it for being an easy road, or that my impairments are gone. Stroke and brain injury will be with me forever, but I am managing it better, a little every day.

It's funny how sometimes incredible things are going on almost right beside us, but we don't notice. I had an event similar to that while I was still working. It was almost like a little bit of foreshadowing for my life now; I have so much chaos inside, but I can keep it well hidden, so most people don't realize it.

Years ago, I was flying back to Edmonton with a co-worker from a work trip to some mines in the USA. We shipped a lot of our product of grinding rods to these mines. The mines used it to crush the raw material and extract iron ore. I left my seat on the plane to use the washroom. While waiting, a man suddenly fell out of the washroom, and it seemed right into my arms. I helped him to the floor while calling out for help. Two flight attendants were there immediately to help me, another paged the cabin to see if a doctor was on board. Luckily the man was breathing and quickly regained consciousness. He had all the help he needed and with so little room, I went back to my seat, without using the washroom. My co-worker asked why I took so long, having no idea about all the commotion. Sometimes there is chaos all around us and we just don't notice it.

Often, now I'm the one just sitting, but I'm aware of the busyness all around me. I can't jump in and help like I used to, like I still want to. We were at Lucy's family's farm for Easter, and I was feeling bad about my lack of help. These were people I knew and loved, but I felt so displaced just sitting there. One of my life teachers suddenly appeared in the form of Lucy's brother. I made a small comment of my frustration but somehow, he understood the depth of my despair. He simply said, "You belong here." I felt tears well up, put my hand on his arm, and said thank you.

UNEXPECTED TEACHERS

Teachers appear in the most unexpected places. Sometimes they offer the most unexpected lessons. My newest teacher of life came in the form of my dental hygienist. We were chatting, or mostly he was as my open mouth made reciprocate conversation impossible. Before he started, I had updated him on my latest stroke and brain surgery. I let him know about the metal plates in my head too, prior to him taking x-rays.

While he was cleaning my teeth, he started musing about the titanium plates in my head. He asked if I had named them. That was something I never even considered. He found the metal plates fascinating and went on, encouraging me to name them, suggesting something like the mutants in X-Men, Magneto or Wolverine. Since I couldn't answer he came up with the name "Excellenium". He was very pleased with the name. Secretly I was too. My hidden mutant X-Man ability, surviving stroke and brain surgery and having four implanted metal plates to prove it, "Excellenium!"

Instead of feeling sorry for me and all that I had been through he changed it into something fun and fantastical. It was another timely lesson. Again, what we see depends on how we look. It made me feel more comfortable. With the gift of good conversation, the hygienist went on. Somehow, he connected my new X-Man name with singing the blues. He felt singing the blues was the right idea for getting problems off your chest.

If you think of any blues songs it is laced with hundreds of problems and is a musical method to express sadness or discouragement. Singing the blues has a long history, originating in the deep south of the USA. Maybe the idea of singing the blues is a way to get your problems out, talk about them or send a message. Sometimes the hardest part is saying it out loud, just like I used to have a hard time telling people I had a stroke.

Once you can say it out loud, you can acknowledge it, address it, and start to move on. You don't have to pretend everything is alright. Bad things happen and sometimes they happen to good people. Start singing your blues and then you can begin to heal, move on. It's like that scene from the movie "Crocodile Dundee" When asked how people deal with problems where he's from in Australia he answer's "…If you got a problem, you tell Wally, and he tells everyone in town. Brings it out in the open, no more problem."

Maybe the dental hygienist was trying to let me know that the best medicine is sometimes just talking openly. Whatever the reason I left the office with clean teeth, no cavities, a spring in my step and a new name for my metal plates; they're my "Excellenium's". They make me excellent because they are a good reminder of what I have survived and even when bad things happen, often there is a gift hidden inside somewhere.

STROKEVERSARY

I celebrated the gift of surviving brain surgery on my one year "Strokeversary". This term was coined by one of my Twitter stroke survivor friends. A Strokeversary is the date you survived your stroke. I have several dates but I'm choosing to celebrate the day I survived brain surgery. My parents came back for another visit and were with Ken and me to celebrate. I'm so appreciative that they take the time and effort to travel and see us. It was a lovely evening and being together enhanced all the reasons I was so grateful.

On the morning of that day, Ken and I took a few moments to ourselves. We got my usual steeped tea and a plain donut from Tim Horton's and went to the beloved Rodeo grounds with Arthur. We just sat together, appreciating the quiet, the calm, the life we could still share together. What a year it had been.

There are times I still miss the old me. The one who would move all the kitchen chairs, turn up the music and dance with the kids, teaching them my novice jive moves. The one who ran Spartan Races just to see how muddy I could get. The one who could climb into railcars, balancing on three-ton bundles of steel bars. The one who could stay up most of the night just to finish a special birthday cake and still have enough energy to host the party. The feelings of loss are getting less and less, replaced with gratitude and hopefully some insight.

I recently had my one year MRI. There was still some residual blood product obscuring the images so the neurosurgeon still couldn't say with certainty if the entire malformation had been removed, but there was nothing new growing or forming. The proverbial sword was there but it was firmly secured. I would continue having regular MRIs to monitor it.

I was also still having appointments with the neuro-ophthalmologist. He still felt my eyes would improve and advised waiting while continuing my eye exercises was the best course. I really wanted my driver's license back. I sorely missed it. I was also realistic about it. Often, I had to close my eyes or look down while Ken was driving. My eyes, or rather, my brain, just couldn't receive and interpret what I was seeing quick enough, and it became a turbulent jumble of colours and unfocused images. I knew I couldn't manage driving on busy roads.

Through stroke and all that has happened I'm learning that most of life happens in multiple shades of gray. I used to be quite black and white; this is wrong, that is right. So many situations in life are tinted with so many tones between pure black and pure white. Just like my imprecise MRI results. Life is teaching me that almost nothing is black or white and I'm learning to find colourful hues within the multitude of grays.

NEWEST GLIA GIRL

Time carried on and finally the illustrations for the newest Glia Girl adventure arrived. They were filled with bright colours and lively action, bringing the story to life. I was excited to start formatting the book. This time Glia Girl helped kids learn about concussion. Concussion can be a huge concern and is finally getting the attention it needs to ensure anyone who experiences one has the time and support to heal properly. I know part of the idea to have Glia Girl explore concussion is because of one of my early childhood experiences.

I remember the incident mostly, but I know my mother remembers it with a clarity I think she would like to forget. I was young, maybe eight or nine. I had gotten a pogo stick and absolutely loved it. I would jump up and down with it, always trying to best the number of bounces I could do without stopping. That day, my parents were working around the house, regular Saturday chores. I was jumping in the garage as my dad had the car pulled out and onto the driveway.

It was perfect jumping grounds, smooth and flat. It felt like I could jump forever when suddenly the bottom of the pogo stick slipped out, the rubber not gripping the smooth concrete. It happened so quickly I had no time to jump off or even react. Thwack! I landed hard, right on the back of my head, right on the hard, unforgiving concrete floor. My mom tells me she still gets the shivers when she thinks about the sound my head hitting the ground made. She rushed me to the doctor.

I seemed okay and the doctor didn't think anything more serious than a concussion had happened. He sent us home with wise words for my mom. Watch me for signs of a worsening head injury, or nausea or excess sleepiness. I'm sure he told her more but that's all I remember. After my first stroke I remember telling the neurologist this story and asking if it could have anything to do with my malformation. He assured me the two were unrelated.

I healed from the concussion, but it scared me. Even my younger self could tell the doctor considered the injury significant. I still sometimes jumped on the pogo stick but no longer with the exuberance I felt before. It took time but the memory of the fall receded, and I found other adventures to fulfill my childhood liveliness.

My own brain injury and old memories of my early concussion spurred the newest *Glia Girl* adventure. With our second *Glia Girl* book out and with COVID-19 becoming endemic, we were ready. Ken started organizing readings at libraries, talks at Senior's Centres, stroke and brain injury support groups, and maybe even some engagements on the radio. I'm quite nervous to be embarking on this new part of our journey but if we can help even one more person, I am fulfilled.

"I slept and dreamt that life was joy. I awoke and saw that life was service. I acted and behold, service was joy." Rabindranath Tagore

CHAPTER 16

LAST CHAPTER – NEW BEGINNINGS

Together Ken and I are embarking on new adventures. He recently retired and I'm so grateful he is using his time to help me in my mission to give back and make the most of my time.

Since my first stroke, giving back and helping others has been my calling. Our podcast, my first book, public speaking engagements all had the common theme of trying to help others and spread information. Stroke can strike at any age, any time.

Often when I tell people I had a stroke I'm met with silence. People don't know what to say. They aren't rude or unkind, they just don't understand. Stroke has such a wide range of outcomes. In TV shows it is usually death or significant disability, but on the flip side, everyone seems to know someone who had a complete recovery and was back at work. My sister Cami suggested I tell people I have a brain injury, maybe that would invite more conversation. Communication is the key first step to understanding.

Ken has good communication skills and is the one with the gift of organization and persuasion. I am so glad he is responsible for calling potential opportunities to promote the books and share my story.

I remember in college, a friend wanted to sell his motorbike. We were visiting when a potential buyer came to look at it. Ken got involved and our friend made more money than he was asking. Our friend's father kept telling everyone that Ken had a "silver tongue". I'm so glad Ken is taking care of contacting people and organizing our schedule. I can write but making phone calls and thinking on the fly like that is something I find challenging.

We still need to be cognizant of my limitations and my health. I can only do so much at a time. I have to be careful where I use up my energies. It is no longer boundless and if I push myself too hard, I pay for it. Ken is right there with me, to help me every step of the way and help me to be the best I can. My mission of giving back and paying it forward has also become his. He is just as grateful for our continued life together.

Life is about change and every experience helps to create the layers that make us who we are. Good, bad, or ugly, they all teach us something. It's up to us to learn the lesson and decide what is important. I've had experiences I never thought I would but that is life, where the unexpected becomes the norm. I've survived unimaginable things. My sister Lydia and I joked one day when recalling all the challenges and kept saying I should title this memoir, "You Can't Make This Shit Up." When I look back at all the things, I am deeply grateful for all I do have. Every situation had the possibility of being so much worse.

The lessons presented to me have influenced how I approach life. There's been many moments when I wanted to stay curled up in a safe cocoon, wrapped in a blanket of sorrow of all I have lost. It might be easier, but this is my life, and it's up to me how I live it. I can't waste the gift that so many people worked hard to give me. My family, my friends, my doctors, the neurosurgeon, the nurses, and healthcare aides, all the different therapists, even my illustrator for the Glia Girl books. There are so many, it would be pages and pages of this memoir to list them all. I am blessed.

So, I'm choosing to make the most of this life. I have been given several second chances. Against the odds, I am still here. I still have gifts to offer, and I have the ability to offer them. I am so fortunate I can still talk and articulate my experiences. I believe I've been given these gifts to try and help others, as I've said before, it's the path I'm meant to be on. I'm trying my hardest.

If sharing my struggles and my story can help someone else to find the strength to make it through another day, I am grateful for my own hardships. When you are going through hard times it can be consuming and overwhelming. During my own I discovered I wasn't alone. Neither are you, dear reader. I feel privileged to share my experiences and honoured that anyone else may find comfort in my words, maybe even the strength to keep going.

We all have a story to tell. Even though our stories may be very different there is always some common thread that binds us together enabling us to find comfort and inspiration and support by sharing. My volunteer work with Covenant Health has really taught me the importance of sharing our stories. Stories bring us together in so many ways. Every story is distinct and unique but even just one thread of commonality and suddenly we are connected.

I recall a breast cancer survivor telling me she had read my first memoir and how she really associated with my experience. She had also lost her career and was living with a sword over her head. Through our very different life altering events we connected and created a bond that remains today. As much as we are bombarded through the news, social media and so many other places, with how different we are, I challenge that we are more alike than we realize. We just need to remember our humanity, find those threads that keep trying to weave us together.

As much as we are unique individuals, we are dependent on one another and sharing our stories is the first step to recognizing our common threads. Let's share, without fear of judgment or prejudice. More importantly, let's listen, with an open heart, recognizing our similarities while celebrating our differences. If we can do that, we are on our way to using all these threads to weave ourselves into a beautiful tapestry called humanity. One where our individual colours and textures can combine to create something new and magnificent, stronger because we have the support of all the other threads surrounding and supporting us, helping us to be our best.

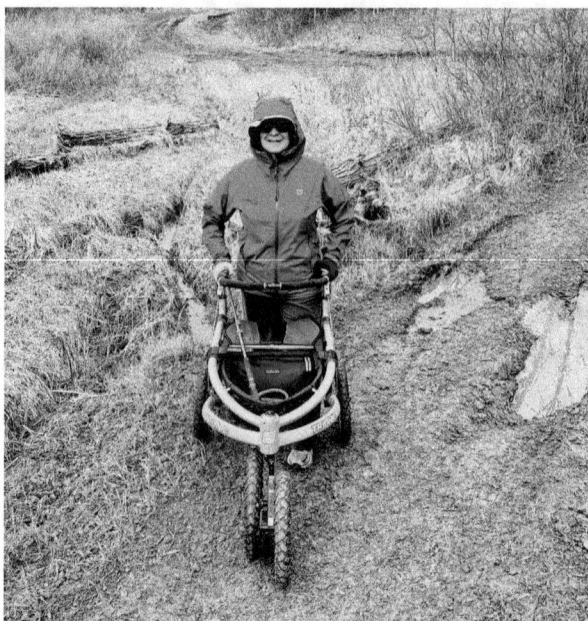

ME AND MY ALL TERRAIN WALKER!

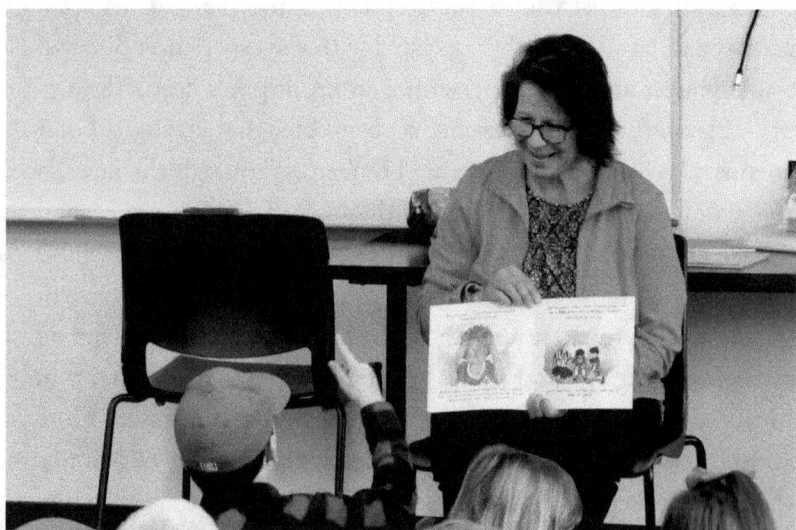

ME READING AN ADVENTURES OF GLIA GIRL
BOOK DURING A LIBRARY PROGRAM.

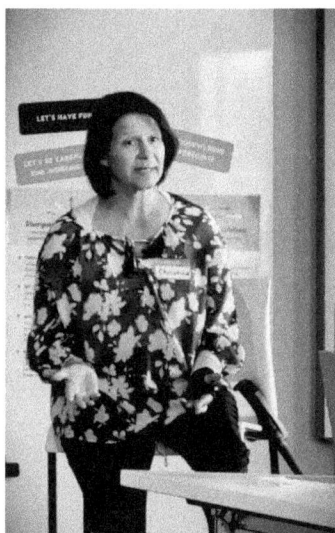

SHARING MY STORY WHEREVER I CAN!

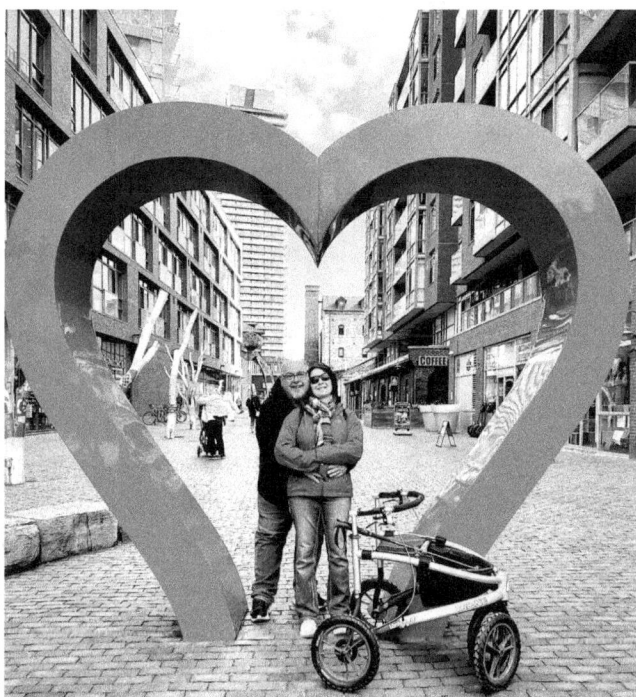

KEN AND I. STILL STRONG DESPITE SO MANY CHALLENGES.

"Life is a journey, a roller coaster ride. When we strip away
fear, we are left with dreams, hopes, and inspiration for a
better tomorrow. Hold onto those. Never Give UP!" CHJ

Epilogue

Moving forward and reaching a point in my own recovery where I can finally really try to help others is the pinnacle of my journey. I recently had my first, and hopefully not my only, television interview, sharing my story, trying to help others. It was scary and exciting. My sister told me instead of letting my nerves get to me, visualize it like waiting to go on a roller coaster ride. She brought it full circle. Life is a roller coaster and I'm trying to help others as much as possible while holding on. I'm also learning to enjoy the ride, not just fear the next loop-de-loop.

As I'm learning to let go of my need for control, I'm also discovering anew that family is so much more than blood relations. I have been blessed with many friends whom I consider family. Family are the people who are there for you, who would drop anything to help you if you were in need. Family answers your calls or texts, share parts of their life with you and are interested in what you are doing. This is caring, this is family. My family is filled with incredible people.

I have so many gold nuggets in my path that I cannot and should not attach my feelings to why some of the things have happened within my own family. I'll say it again for I feel it is so important. Whenever a life altering event happens to one person, ensure everyone has the support needed to navigate the turbulent waters of life's tribulations. The survivor is the captain of the boat, but all the passengers are affected too.

Every day I try to find goodness and express appreciation for what I have. I'm choosing to live a grateful life. All these experiences have contributed to my outlook on life and hopefully awarded me some wisdom. I am much more compassionate to those I encounter. My own invisible challenges remind me to not judge others. They may be smiling, interacting, and trying to live their best life but who knows what torment they are trying to manage on the inside. I have no right to judge, only to extend whatever understanding and compassion I can.

To my dear future reader, I hope by the time you are reading my story, my bucket list has been fulfilled. I hope my family is reunited, but there is so much more to my life. Long have I travelled on this road of surviving multiple strokes, prevailing through brain surgery, and continuously striving to live my best life on a path of ever changing normal. Through this crazy roller coaster ride called life I have discovered I am grateful for my challenges and my survival, for the chance to help others in ways I would have never considered without my journey.

Just a few more Words:

I am so lucky to still be alive, to be here for everyone I love and care for. I am so grateful for my life and the many teachers who have appeared throughout my journey, patiently waiting for me to learn my lessons, to soak up the wisdom offered, and then share it, using my experiences to help others. I am appreciating each and every day, focusing on the present, stopping to consider life events as lessons instead of ignoring them because I am focusing on tomorrow.

I'm still here doing what I'm doing because my cloak of love and support helping me every step of the way is snugly wrapped around my shoulders. My goal is to create a circle. I envision standing hand in hand with other survivors, telling our stories, sharing our struggles, our successes, lending our strength to one another. My success belongs to all who have helped weave the fabric of my cloak. I know I am not alone. I am forever grateful. I feel I have grown and learned enough where I have the honour of hopefully being a thread in someone else's cloak.

"I hope you will go out and let stories, ... happen to you, and that you will work with these stories... water them with your blood and tears and your laughter till they bloom, till you yourself burst into bloom."
C. Pinkola Estes, Women Who Run with Wolves

Thank you for completing *I Am Alive*.

We would love if you could help by posting a review at your book retailer and on the PageMaster Publishing site. It only takes a minute and it would really help others by giving them an idea of your experience.

Thanks

7jarsofhotpickledpeppers.com

Christine Holubec-Jackson at the PageMaster store
https://pagemasterpublishing.ca/by/christine-holubec-jackson/

To order more copies of this book, find books by other Canadian authors, or make inquiries about publishing your own book, contact PageMaster at:

PageMaster Publication Services Inc.
11340-120 Street, Edmonton, AB T5G 0W5
books@pagemaster.ca
780-425-9303

catalogue and e-commerce store
PageMasterPublishing.ca/Shop